WITH ALL MY
HEART

God's Design for Emotional Wellness

by Paul Carlisle, Ph.D.

LifeWay Press
Nashville, Tennessee

ISBN 0-6330-0583-5

Dewey Decimal Classification: 152.4
Subject Heading: EMOTIONS\MENTAL HEALTH

This book is the text for courses CG-0535 in the Personal Life area in the Christian Growth Study Plan.

Unless otherwise noted, Scripture quotations are taken from the Holy Bible,
New International Version, copyright © 1973, 1978, 1984
by International Bible Society.

Scripture quotations identified NKJV are from the *New King James Version.*
Copyright © 1979, 1980, 1982, Thomas Nelson, Inc. Publishers. Used by permission.

Scripture quotations identified KJV are from the *King James Version.*

Scripture quotations identified NLT are from the Holy Bible, *New Living Translation,*
copyright © 1996. Used by permission of Tyndale House Publishers, Inc., Wheaton, Illinois 60189.
All rights reserved.

To order additional copies of this resource: WRITE LifeWay Church Resources Customer Service,
127 Ninth Avenue, North, Nashville, TN 37234-0113; FAX order to (615) 251-5933;
PHONE 1-800-458-2772; EMAIL to *customerservice@lifeway.com*; ONLINE at *www.lifeway.com;*
or visit the LifeWay Christian Store serving you.

For information about adult discipleship and family resources, training, and events,
visit our Web site at *www.lifeway.com/discipleplus.*

For information about Fit 4, visit our Web site at *www.fit4.com.*

Printed in the United States of America.

LifeWay Press
127 Ninth Avenue, North
Nashville, Tennessee 37234-0151

*As God works through us, we will help people and churches know Jesus Christ and seek His kingdom
by providing biblical solutions that spiritually transform individuals and cultures.*

Branda Polk, Health Ministry Specialist
Betty Hassler, Editor
Jon Rodda, Art Director
Jimmy Abegg, Illustrator
Joyce McGregor, Assistant Editor
Rhonda Porter Delph, Manuscript Assistant

Table of Contents

AN INTRODUCTION TO *Fit4*

With All My Heart: God's Design for Emotional Wellness is one of four continuing studies in *Fit 4: A Life Way Christian Wellness Plan.* If this is your first *Fit 4* study, welcome to this series which helps individuals achieve wellness one wise choice at a time. Wellness is a lifestyle which includes all four areas of our lives: emotional, spiritual, mental, and physical.

Although this study emphasizes emotional wellness, the other areas of wellness are referred to throughout the book because whole-person health involves all that we are. Jesus said it best in Mark 12:30-31—the *Fit 4* theme verses— when he outlined a wellness lifestyle: "Love the Lord your God with all your heart and with all your soul and with all your mind and with all your strength. Love your neighbor as yourself."

Fit 4 emphasizes three Lifestyle Disciplines to help you live a balanced lifestyle. UPREACH is your relationship to God through daily prayer, Bible reading, and listening to God. OUTREACH is your relationship with others. INREACH is caring for yourself mentally, emotionally, physically, and spiritually. Each week of this study you will find information in the margins which will give you practical suggestions for implementing each of these discplines daily.

Since our emotions are housed in a body which requires proper food and nutrition to function properly, you will also find in each week a helpful suggestion from our friend Professor Phitt, one of the hosts in the *Fit 4* videos that accompany the two basic courses. These suggestions, found in the margin of each week's reading, will guide you as you make wise choices in exercise and nutrition.

fit 4
heart • soul • mind • strength
A LIFEWAY CHRISTIAN WELLNESS PLAN

Your *Accountability Journal* will be your friend on your wellness journey. On pages 6-10 you will find information on how to use the *Journal* to track your exercise and food choices for the next 12 weeks. Record your exercise to see patterns, make changes, and set goals to improve your fitness level. Record the food you eat so you become aware of the types and amounts of your daily choices. For more information on making these wise choices, consult pages 14-22 of your *Journal.*

Your group will support your wellness journey. While you encourage and support others, they will do the same for you. Your facilitator will also encourage you as you journey toward emotional wellness. Plan to be present for each group session. Contribute your ideas, ask questions, and seek answers from other group members' struggles, victories, and life experiences.

For additional information on a wellness lifestyle, consider being part of a *Fit 4* basic course. *Fit 4 Nutrition* is a 12-week course that will help you apply the *Fit 4* Guidelines for Healthy Eating. *Fit 4 Fitness* is a 12-week course that will help you develop your own personalized fitness plan.

You will also want to participate in the other three continuing studies: *With All My Soul: God's Design for Spiritual Wellness,* 0-6330-0585-1; *With All My Mind: God's Design for Mental Wellness,* 06330-0584-3; and *With All My Strength: God's Design for Physical Wellness,* 0-6330-0586-X. Information about how to order these and other *Fit 4* resources is found on page 95.

ABOUT THE AUTHOR

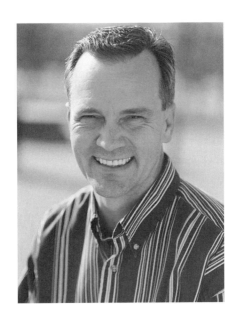

Dr. Paul Carlisle is Professor of Pastoral Counseling and Care at Midwestern Baptist Theological Seminary in Kansas City, Missouri. Paul is the co-author of *Strength for the Journey: A Biblical Perspective on Discouragement and Depression* (LifeWay Press, 1999). He is also a conference leader and writer with a passion for spiritual transformation and mentoring.

Paul is a member of the *Fit 4* Advisory Panel and is featured on both the *Nutrition* and *Fitness* group session videos. He is married to Terri and they have two children, Chase and Chelsea. Paul enjoys leisure reading and watching and playing basketball.

ABOUT THE STUDY

With All My Heart: God's Design for Emotional Wellness is intended as a group study over a 12-week period. The first week's group session will give you an overview of *Fit 4: A LifeWay Christian Wellness Plan.* During this session, you will complete the video viewer guide on page 6.

During the following 10 weeks, you will read each week's content and complete the learning activities which are marked with the *Fit 4* logo. Read the week's material at your own pace. Make sure you complete the reading before the weekly group session. The learning activities provide practice and review for the concepts you will learn. They also improve retention of what you read. A Verse to Know at the beginning of each week will enable you to commit to memory specific verses which will aid you in your wellness journey.

In the margins you will read suggestions for implementing the three Lifestyle Disciplines of *Fit 4:* UPREACH, OUTREACH, INREACH. You will also find

helpful advice from our friend Professor Phitt, one of the video hosts from the *Fit 4* basic courses. Professor Phitt will give suggestions for exercise and nutrition choices. The *Accountability Journal* accompanying this book will also encourage you in your wellness journey.

A Leader Guide on pages 88-94 provides the group facilitator with specific information for beginning and conducting a class using *With All My Heart: God's Design for Emotional Wellness.*

Week 12 of this study is a group session which provides an opportunity for members to evaluate progress toward goals, set new goals for maintaining a wellness lifestyle, and make plans for participating in other *Fit 4* or discipleship studies.

Remember our *Fit 4* motto: Wellness is achieved one wise choice at a time.

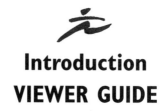

Introduction
VIEWER GUIDE

1. *Fit 4* is designed to help you develop a _____ approach to wellness.

2. What is wellness?

3. The secret to good health is _____.

4. You will use the *Fit 4* guidelines to develop a _____ plan to meet your needs.

5. What is the purpose of your *Fit 4* group?

6. What is the role of your *Fit 4* facilitator?

7. Who is Professor Phitt?

8. Why is seeking wellness important to your relationship with God?

9. What are the Lifestyle Disciplines of *Fit 4?* U_____, O_____, and I_____.

10. Based on what you know thus far, list some personal benefits you can expect to gain from completing this study.

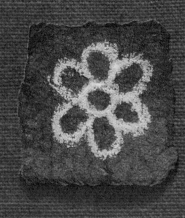

Week One
Emotions: Vital Part of Total Wellness

Ask a few friends, *What are emotions?* and you will get a wide variety of answers. My research indicates that the word *emotion* does not have an agreed-upon definition. We need to begin our study of emotions by mapping out the terrain. Like Lewis and Clark, we are going into uncharted territory; watch your step!

Emotional wellness is integrally related to mental, physical, and spiritual wellness. All four aspects must work together for balanced, whole-person health. Picture a chest with four drawers. Each drawer contains a different item of clothing; yet it takes all four items to be completely clothed. So it is with emotional wellness. The "emotional wellness drawer" in your life chest may be filled to the brim and neat as a pin. But without the other three drawers—mental, spiritual, and physical wellness—you will not experience total wellness. We are whole persons.

Although this study opens up only one of the four drawers for close inspection, we are not dismissing the physical, mental, and spiritual drawers. You will find suggestions in the margins for activities that encourage whole-person health. These suggestions are based on the *Lifestyle Disciplines of **Fit 4**: A LifeWay Christian Wellness Plan* (see p. 4): **UPREACH, OUTREACH,** and **INREACH.**

In the margins you will also find tips from Professor Phitt—one of the **Fit4** video hosts—on healthy eating and exercise. Our emotions don't exist in a vacuum. They live in a body that is fueled by the food we eat and physically fit according to our exercise routine. Emotions are also influenced by thought patterns and by spiritual input. You will profit from learning the Verse to Know each week. As you meditate on God's Word, you will grow in your capacity to see God's perspective—one of the keys to emotional balance. Let's begin our study of emotional wellness by asking, *How are our emotions affected by our bodies?*

EMOTIONS ARE PHYSICAL

Emotions in their simplest form are biological: they cannot be separated from the marvelously complex body God provided for you.

VERSES TO KNOW

" 'Love the Lord your God with all your heart and with all your soul and with all your mind and with all your strength.' The second is this: 'Love your neighbor as yourself.' "
—Mark 12:30-31

Getting a yearly physical exam is one way we take good care of our emotions. Our physical well-being influences our emotional well-being. If you have not scheduled your annual physical, do so today.

The Brain

The human brain plays an important role in the body's experiencing and expressing emotions. The cognitive (thinking) and emotional (feeling) aspects of the brain are so interrelated that they cannot be separated. In other words, the brain does not separate feelings from facts or facts from feelings. Some researchers conclude that feelings are merely psychological and neurological arousal attached to facts.[1]

Does the statement that the brain does not separate fact from feeling surprise you? (Check one.) ❑ Yes ❑ No

Thoughts and feelings may be more inter-connected than you realized.

Body Chemicals

John Medina explains the role of body chemicals in the way we experience emotions, especially depression. "Chemicals exist in our brains which help it to function properly. Some of these chemicals can mediate how we feel emotionally. A proper balance of these substances is important for maintaining normal well-adjusted lives. Modern research has discovered that depression is associated with an imbalance of some of these brain chemicals. This imbalance can occur because of environmental inputs, self-defeating thinking, or even faulty genetic wiring."[2]

Dr. Dwight Carlson, a Christian psychiatrist, contends, "The evidence for a biological basis for some emotional illnesses has grown so great that to consider them as different from physical illnesses can no longer be justified."[3] He cites the example of lack of light, which can cause depression in some people. This condition is called *seasonal affective disorder (S.A.D.)* and is biological in origin.[4]

Stress

Archibald Hart, a seminary professor, relates emotions and stress. "The word stress means different things to different people. It ... includes changes in perception, emotions, behavior, and physical functioning. Some think of it only as tension, others as anxiety. Some think of it as good, others as bad. The truth is that we all need a certain amount of stress to keep us alive, although too much of it becomes harmful to us."[5]

Hart explains that stress plays a role in bodily sickness "by destroying the body's immunological defense mechanism. In other words, too much stress saps the body's ability to fight off disease, so that viruses and bacteria thrive. ...The process takes place slowly, eventually robbing us of just enough 'fighting power' to place us at jeopardy for illness. There is even some suspicion that stress may cause some forms of cancer to grow more rapidly because the body's ability to fight off the growth of cancerous cells is destroyed or diminished."[6]

Dr. Hart points out some general symptoms of excessive stress that are emotional in nature: feelings of "trembling," fear of impending doom, feelings of fatigue and lack of energy or heaviness, heightened irritability and anger, racing thoughts, daydreaming, indecisiveness, and sleep disruption.[7]

We were created in such a way that our bodies impact the way we experience emotions. For example, diabetics, whose blood sugar levels fluctuate, experience intense swings of emotions. Can you remember a time when you had a severe case of the flu or a similar sickness? Do you remember your emotional state? In my case, my emotions reflected the state of my body. I felt uncomfortable, discouraged, irritable, and tired. Your body has a definite impact on your emotions.

 Recall a very happy time in your life. Was your health generally good? (Check one.) ❑ Yes ❑ No
Now think of a particularly stressful memory. Do you recall any health concerns? ❑ Yes ❑ No
If yes, would you say your health was generally which of the following? (Check one.) ❑ poor ❑ average ❑ good
As you experienced less stress, did your health improve? (Check one.) ❑ Yes ❑ No

Food Intake

Have you ever had such a busy day that you did not take time to eat? What do you remember feeling as hunger set in? Did you feel irritable? grouchy? fatigued? impatient? Food intake has a direct impact on how you feel. Food is your body's energy source. Without it your body short-circuits much like a hair dryer that is dropped into a tub of water. Unlike the hair dryer, you do not have an obvious indicator of short-circuited emotions. You do not smoke and spark like the hair dryer, but both of you are damaged. If you had such obvious signals, you would probably quickly address your need for food.

 Eating some foods may evoke certain emotions. Check which emotion(s) you might feel when consuming the following:

	PLEASURE	DISGUST	EXCITEMENT	BOREDOM
Buttered popcorn	❑	❑	❑	❑
Liver	❑	❑	❑	❑
Hot fudge sundae	❑	❑	❑	❑
Fried chicken	❑	❑	❑	❑
Sardines	❑	❑	❑	❑
Hamburger	❑	❑	❑	❑
Prime rib	❑	❑	❑	❑
Brussels sprouts	❑	❑	❑	❑
Potatoes	❑	❑	❑	❑

Rest

The man and his wife had shocked looks on their faces. The couple had come to my counseling office at the suggestion of their pastor and were prepared to do whatever it took to improve their marriage: deepen intimacy, practice communication skills, or read books on conflict resolution. I suppose that is why they were shocked when I suggested that more sleep would greatly improve their marriage. I understood their skepticism. What person would consider sleep as a major factor in the success of life or marriage?

"As water reflects a face, so a man's heart reflects the man."
—Proverbs 27:19

INREACH
Think about the emotions you feel at those times when you may eat too much or too little. Compare them with your emotions when you have consumed only as much food as you really need. Record emotional responses to food under "Thoughts for the Day" in your *Accountability Journal*.

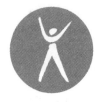

UPREACH

Exodus 20:8 says,
"Remember the Sabbath day
by keeping it holy."

Obeying this commandment
is in your best interest. Make
a commitment to begin or
continue practicing
a day of rest.

"Stand at the crossroads and
look; ...
ask where the good way is, and
walk in it,
and you will find rest."
—Jeremiah 6:16

The amount of rest we get greatly influences our emotional control. I believe that what I suggested to the couple about their need for rest is true for all of us. Below are some facts about the importance of rest.

1. Societal pressures to work more and at odd hours have reduced our sleep time over the past century by about 20 percent.[8] People are driven to have and to do it all—work, family, sports, hobbies—and there is very little time left for rest.

2. Every day sleepy people make math errors, break things, and become cross with their families, friends, and coworkers. They make mistakes with tragic consequences. It is hard to prove how many fatal car accidents are caused by drivers' falling asleep, but researchers believe the number is high.

3. Researchers believe that too little sleep results in sleep debt. Like monetary debt, sleep debt must be paid back! If you get an hour less than a full night's sleep, you carry an hour of sleep debt into the next day.

4. Sickness may be one way your body pays off sleep debt. As a matter of fact, accumulated sleep debt may do long-term damage to your health. For example, the American Cancer society surveyed over one million Americans about their exercise, nutrition, smoking, sleep, and other habits. After tracking the group for six years, they found that short sleep time had a high correlation with mortality. If people had originally reported sleeping less than seven hours a night, they were far more likely to be dead within six years than those who slept an average of seven hours per night.[9]

5. One of the major effects of sleep deprivation is mood swings. People who get less than a full night's sleep are prone to feel less happy, more stressed, more physically frail, and more mentally and physically exhausted. Lowering sleep debt can make us feel better, happier, more vigorous, and vital.

6. You can't work off a large sleep debt by getting a good night's sleep. You have to make up as much sleep as possible and avoid amassing another large sleep debt by adopting a sleep-smart lifestyle.

7. Most people are poor judges of whether they are getting enough rest. Only about two out of ten people are aware of whether they get sufficient rest.[10]

Lack of sleep has a tremendous impact on emotional health and physical well-being. God made us with a need for regular rest and stillness. He established regular weekly periods of rest for the Israelites through Sabbath observance. God knew people needed one day a week to recover from daily activity, not a couple of weeks of vacation a year. If we followed Sabbath observance, we would get 52 days off a year. God knows how our bodies work best. When we follow His plan, we can maximize our service for Him all our lives.

Read Jeremiah 6:16 in the margin. How does Jeremiah say we find rest? Underline it.

Exercise

Another indicator of the body's relationship to our feelings is exercise. Medical science is convinced of the emotional benefit of working out, especially aerobic exercise. (See *Fit4 Fitness Member Workbook*.) Stress and negative emotions accumulate throughout our day because of work and family pressures much like a sink serves as a collector of dirty dishes. If your family is like mine, we have a choice when it comes to dirty dishes. We can let them pile (we have yet to reach the ceiling, but we have come close on several occasions!), or we can roll up our sleeves and wash them by hand or place them in the dishwasher. The results are a sink ready to handle more dirty dishes the next day. Stress and negative emotions pile up like dirty dishes. Exercise is a common activity every person can use to begin eliminating the accumulated negative emotions. The exercise can be as simple as a brisk walk or as structured as treadmills or resistance training. The choice is yours! The benefits will be immeasurable for you and those you love.

EMOTIONS ARE SPIRITUAL

Our emotions are an important part of our faith. Recall your salvation experience. Clearly fix that moment in your mind. Do you remember the place? Were there other people around, or were you by yourself? Can you recall what you felt?

I was about 16, sitting on the back seat of a small country church. I was a bit anxious before I made the decision to accept Jesus as my Savior and Lord. After opening my heart to the Savior, I felt peace and joy. All was well. I knew the Master.

Trusting Christ for salvation has an emotional component that cannot be denied. The Christian life is spiritual, mental, physical, and emotional. We damage our spiritual life if we attempt to disregard any of the four. Next week we will examine God's emotional makeup. We are like God. It is only reasonable to expect that we would be emotional beings as well as spiritual beings.

 Read Psalm 100 in the margin. Underline the various emotions that are mentioned.

EMOTIONS ARE MENTAL

What you *think* has an impact on what you *believe you can do*. For instance, if you continually tell yourself you can't do a particular task such as water-skiing, then there is a very good chance that you will not be successful. Sports psychologists have the challenging job of helping athletes perform at higher levels. They teach them to restructure their thinking in more positive ways. When a basketball player misses a shot, he is instructed to tell himself he will do better next time rather than saying to himself, "That was a horrible shot." Sports psychologists understand the mind-body relationship.

Let's look at how this process worked in Numbers 13–14. The Israelites faced a formidable foe. The spies gave a majority report that the land was good, the people in the land were strong, and the cities were large and fortified (13:28). The encounter left the 10 spies thinking, "We are not able to go up against the people, for they are stronger than we" (v. 31, NKJV). They concluded, "we were like grasshoppers in our own sight, and so we were in their sight" (v. 33, NKJV). This report led to intense weeping (strong emotions) in the Israelite camp (14:1).

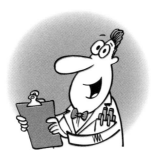

Professor Phitt says:
If you do not have an exercise plan, begin by walking 20 minutes three times a week. Choose a safe place to walk, such as your neighborhood, a gym, or a local mall.

"Shout for joy to the Lord,
    all the earth.
  Worship the Lord with
    gladness;
  come before him with
    joyful songs.
Know that the Lord is God.
  It is he who made us, and
    we are his;
we are his people, the sheep
  of his pasture.
Enter his gates with
    thanksgiving
  and his courts with praise;
  give thanks to him and
    praise his name.
For the Lord is good and his
    love endures forever;
  his faithfulness continues
    through all generations."
  —Psalm 100

The Israelites began to express frustration and anger about their decision to leave Egypt. Some even wanted to stone Moses, select another leader, and return home. As I read this account, I realized that the Israelites were paralyzed with fear, yet there was not one enemy in their midst. Although there was no real threat, their thoughts alone produced intense anxiety. What you think has a tremendous impact on what you feel. In chapter 7 you will find strategies to help you think in ways that produce healthy feelings.

This same relationship between the mind and body is true for emotions. What we believe has tremendous impact on what we feel and what we do. Look at the chart on page 13 which provides a simple diagram of how thinking impacts emotions.

Apply to your life this process on page 13. You will identify how thoughts and emotions affect how you feel and what you do.

EMOTIONS ARE RELATIONAL

Emotions are the voice of relationships. Emotions function like a doppler radar. They constantly update us on the status of our relationships. They detect a relational storm building and quickly report it to us via feelings. Our emotions provide a portable radar screen that we can check occasionally to see how we are handling our relationships. Although our emotions serve as a portable radar screen, often they are hidden or obscured. We do not always have a clear picture. Sometimes emotions result from too little input. We make leaps in our logic to fill in the gaps. Recognize that emotions can be inaccurate and allow for such.

Relationships can be divided into three categories: 1) relationship to God, 2) relationship to others, and 3) relationship to self. Recall that these are the three *Lifestyle Disciplines of Fit 4*—**UPREACH, OUTREACH,** and **INREACH**—based on your Verse(s) to Know for this week. Reread the verses printed on page 7. God's Word reveals how emotions connect to these three types of relationships.

Read the following Scripture passages in your Bible. Beside each verse identify the emotion(s) in the passage and check whether the verse refers to our relationship to God, others, or oneself (the person speaking).

	Emotion(s)	GOD	SELF	OTHERS
Genesis 1:31	_____	❑	❑	❑
Psalm 40:12	_____	❑	❑	❑
1 John 4:20	_____	❑	❑	❑

These are some examples of how emotions and relationships interact. I have not been able to find one single Bible verse where emotions are reported and not connected to a relationship to God, others, or self. Emotions are always to be understood in the context of these three relationships.

OUTREACH

As you study emotional wellness over the next nine weeks, think about how your emotional expression affects others in your circle of influence—family, friends, coworkers, and neighbors.

THE STRESS MODEL

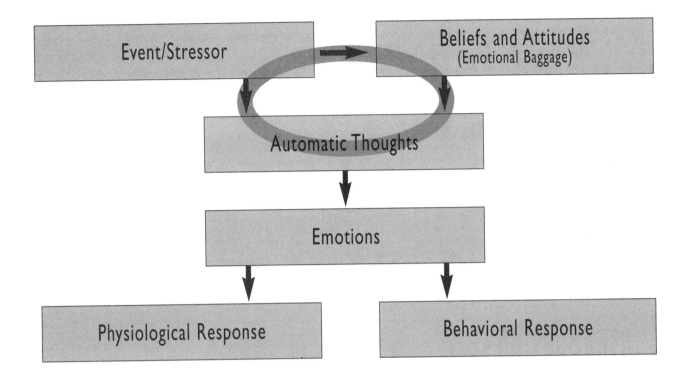

This diagram, adapted from one used at the Mind/Body Medical Institute at Harvard*, shows us how stress works its way into our lives. As **events** come into our awareness, they may or may not become **stressors**. Whether they become stressors depends on the interaction between the event and our personal history, something we can think of as our **beliefs and attitudes** or simply as "emotional baggage." Everyone has baggage! Each individual's baggage is the sum total of the beliefs and attitudes developed in response to past events in his or her life. Some baggage is useful—if you put your hand on a hot stove, it will burn you. Some no longer serves a purpose—if I cross the street without holding someone's hand, I may be hit by a car. Often we continue to hold onto emotional baggage even after it no longer serves us.

Events that take place interact with our beliefs and attitudes and lead to **automatic thoughts**—the unconscious thoughts we have all day long. The majority of our thoughts tend to be negative simply because they try to help us prepare for whatever might happen to us. They

also open us to potentially distorted thoughts. Thoughts lead to **emotions**. Emotions are biochemical and physiological as well as mental. These biochemical changes can lead to **physiological** changes that we call stress. They also produce **behavioral** responses.

Notice that **thoughts precede emotions** and that emotions are biochemical changes in your body. This process sets up a cycle or loop in which your mind identifies the biochemical events and labels them as an emotion. Certain biochemical changes may be identified as anger, sadness, happiness, or joy—but the point is that thought precedes emotions. Think happy thoughts, experience happy emotions. Think angry thoughts, feel anger.

Because we each have the ability to change our thoughts, we can change how we feel. We are not helpless victims of our emotions. We have power that we can choose to exercise. Abraham Lincoln has been quoted as saying, "Most people are about as happy as they make up their minds to be." He was right.

* Adapted from Herbert Benson, M.D., and Eileen Stuart, R.N.C., M.S., *The Wellness Book: The Comprehensive Guide to Maintaining Health and Treating Stress-Related Illness* (New York: Simon & Schuster, 1993).

> " 'Are not two sparrows sold for a penny? Yet not one of them will fall to the ground apart from the will of your Father. And even the very hairs of your head are all numbered. So don't be afraid; you are worth more than many sparrows.' "
> —Matthew 10:29-31

EMOTIONS ARE!

This week we have attempted to determine how emotions relate to our bodies, minds, and spirits. Emotions are the product of biology, thoughts, and relationships. Emotions are an important way we express our spiritual lives. Emotions are complex and multifaceted and will never be explained adequately in simple terms. Most importantly, emotions just are! Since they are a vital part of who God created us to be, let's thank God for making us emotional beings. Pray the following prayer along with me, or write one of your own in the margin.

> *Father, this week I have been reminded of Your marvelous creative abilities. Understanding all the components of my emotional makeup is beyond me. But I know You understand all things about me. You are the one who knows when a sparrow falls. Now teach me to know You in my inner being, that I may reflect You in all of my life—especially my emotions. Amen.*

Explain in your own words the relationship between our emotional, spiritual, mental, and physical selves.

_____

_____

_____

_____

[1] William T. Kirwan, *Biblical Concepts for Christian Counseling* (Grand Rapids, MI: Baker Book House, 1984), 49-50.
[2] John Medina, *Depression: How It Happens!* (Hong Kong; CME, Inc., 1998), 32.
[3] Dwight L. Carlson, M.D., *Why Do Christians Shoot Their Wounded?* (Downer's Grove, IL: InterVarsity Press, 1994), 75.
[4] Ibid., 84.
[5] Archibald Hart, *Adrenalin and Stress* (Dallas: Word Publishing, 1991), 4.
[6] Ibid., 7.
[7] Ibid., 55.
[8] William C. Dement, M.D., and Christopher Vaughan, "Getting Enough Sleep," *Reader's Digest,* September 1999, 112-117.
[9] Ibid.
[10] Ibid.
[11] Robert S. McGee, *Search for Significance* (Nashville: LifeWay Press, 1998), 214.

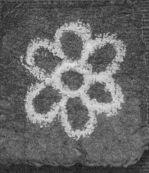

Why Do We Have Emotions?

VERSE TO KNOW

"So God created man in his
    own image,
  in the image of God he
    created him;
  male and female he created
    them."
          —Genesis 1:27

When you look in the mirror, can you isolate the source of your emotions? Where do they come from and why do you have them? The Bible does not explain the source or nature of emotions, nor does it attempt to explain how emotions are influenced by life experiences. The Bible assumes the reality and variety of emotions—both for God and all humankind.

As I prepared to write this study, I began surveying familiar Bible passages looking for expressions of emotion. To my surprise, they covered nearly every page of the Bible. I was even more surprised to discover the rich variety of emotions attributed to God. This week we will examine some of the emotions of God recorded in the Bible. Perhaps you are asking, *What do God's emotions have to do with me?*

HOW DO GOD'S EMOTIONS RELATE TO YOU?

In a classic scene from the movie "The Christmas Story," two boys argued on a school playground during recess. One boy believed tongues didn't stick to frozen metal, and the other boy angrily stated that tongues did stick to frozen metal. Everyone crowded around as these two verbally "duked" it out. One boy's dare became a double-dog-dare. All the boys knew that the double-dog-dare required the other party to prove it. When the recess bell sounded, the little boy who took the dare was left in the playground alone, his tongue stuck to the metal pole.

Unlike the boys in the movie, I am in no way issuing a double-dog-dare, but I am issuing a challenge. Are you willing to tackle the subject of God's emotions? Some believers shy away from any discussion of emotions, especially God's. Others place little emphasis upon this aspect of His personhood. I want you to join me in recognizing the significance of God as an emotional Being. By the way, this will be much less painful than having your tongue stuck to a frozen metal pole.

 Does the fact that God is an emotional Being affect you? Do His emotions ever impact your life? Circle a phrase to indicate your opinion.

has no impact at all   has some impact   has a lot of impact

HOW IS GOD EMOTIONAL?

As I studied passages where God interacted with humans, I was amazed at the variety of emotions exhibited by our Creator.

Divine Sadness

Sadness is a common emotion that may result from an unhappy encounter with another person or may occur simply because we are human. We feel sad because our favorite team lost, the electric bill was so high, or we broke our glasses.

Because God is perfection, He does not experience sadness due to His own frailty or miscalculations. However, our God allows Himself to be touched by our lives. In Genesis 6:6 God reacted with painful emotions to the wickedness of the people. Being rejected by those He created wounded the heart of our Creator.

> "He was grieved
> in His heart."
> —Genesis 6:6 (NKJV)

The New Testament offers us another picture of God's sadness. Jesus, the second Person of the Trinity, was with dear friends whose brother had died. He spoke with the sisters and—looking at Mary grieving—Jesus "groaned in the spirit, and was troubled" (John 11:33, KJV). Then he began to weep (v. 35). Do you get the significance of this picture? Jesus our Savior was overcome with sadness and grief. Although He knew that Mary's brother Lazarus was going to be raised from the dead, He cried because He was touched by Mary's grief.

Read Matthew 23:37-39 for another glimpse of our Savior experiencing sadness. Jesus had just confronted the religious leaders with their unwillingness to follow Him. Jesus lamented, " 'O Jerusalem, Jerusalem, you who kill the prophets and stone those sent to you, how often I have longed to gather your children together, as a hen gathers her chicks under her wings, but you were not willing' " (v. 37). What a phenomenal word-picture! The hen and chicks symbolize Jesus' desire to be close and nurturing to those who had just rejected and condemned Him. What saddened the heart of our Savior was the unwillingness of the people of Jerusalem to draw near to Him. This is a vivid picture of the God-Man, Jesus, reacting with sadness to the rejection of others.

> "Do not grieve the
> Holy Spirit of God."
> —Ephesians 4:30

The third Person of the Trinity also experiences sadness. In the margin, read what Paul said about the Holy Spirit. The apostle told the believers at Ephesus that their lives could impact God the Holy Spirit in such a way as to cause Him sadness.

These passages reveal that God the Father, God the Son, and God the Holy Spirit all feel sadness. Our God is touched by our lives. We call Jesus *Immanuel* because He is with us (Matt. 1:23). God allows us such a close relationship with Him that the condition of our hearts and our actions touch His heart.

 Ask God to reveal how you touch His heart. Spend some time in prayer. Thank God for caring about your pain and the sadness your and others' sin brings into your life. Thank Him for His forgiveness when you grieve the Holy Spirit. Thank God for the new start He provides each day.

Heavenly Happiness

He danced around the delivery room with his hands held high. Every expression said, "I am ecstatic!" Then he danced up and down the hospital hallways, telling everyone he saw that he was a new father. Life is peppered with pictures of happiness—a child graduating from school or scoring the winning goal, a promotion at work, a hug from a grandchild, or a special gift from someone you love.

We are accustomed to thinking of humans as happy, but thinking of God as happy may be a new concept for you. It certainly was for me. I recall a time when I did not think of God in positive emotional terms. Yet in His Word God experiences happiness often.

The minor prophet Zephaniah recorded for us a time when God experienced extreme happiness. Zephaniah was writing to a people who needed to turn back to God and would soon be taken into Babylonian captivity. In the margin read the prophet's record of these astonishing words.

These words took me by surprise. The possibility of God rejoicing over His people—or me—was too marvelous! I always thought God endured me, but now I was confronted with the idea of His enjoying me! What a shock! Believing that God experiences happiness is one thing, but believing that I could be the reason for His happiness is awesome.

God's view of His relationship with me is quite different from my own. I matter to God, and so do you. In the Zephaniah passage, God is happy in relationship to us.

Think of a recent time when you brought God happiness. Oh, come on, don't be modest. I imagine He was happy when you opened this book!

_____

_____

Holy Anger

What emotion do you most often associate with God? For me the answer is easy: anger. As a young teen, I had no doubt in my adolescent mind about God being "mad." It pains me that I embraced this unfair and imbalanced view of our Heavenly Father, but I imagine that I am not alone in having had this view of God.

Have you ever felt God was mostly angry? At what time in your life? Why did you experience Him as angry?

_____

_____

"On that day they will say to
   Jerusalem,
   Do not fear, O Zion;
   do not let your hands hang
      limp.
The Lord your God is with you,
   he is mighty to save.
He will take great delight
      in you,
   he will quiet you with
      his love,
he will rejoice over you with
      singing.' "
      —Zephaniah 3:16-17

INREACH

Research has linked chronic anger with the potential for heart disease. If you find yourself feeling angry on a regular basis, consider the consequences. Anger should be a response to a particular life event, not a lifestyle.

Anger is definitely part of God's emotional make-up. Let's peek into the Book of Exodus for a clear picture of God expressing anger. The scene is the wilderness of Sinai where on the mountain in a face-to-face encounter with God, Moses received the Ten Commandments. Back at the camp, the Israelites tired of Moses' absence and made a golden calf to soothe their worship-hunger. God instructed Moses to come down from the mountain because the people's hearts had turned to an idol. Exodus 32:10 says that in His anger God intended to destroy the children of Israel and make a nation out of Moses' descendants. Only Moses' intercession turned away God's wrath from the Israelites. Why was God angry? Was it because the Israelites had defected, or because they were choosing a way of life that would ultimately destroy them? The answer may be some of both. It is abundantly clear that God expressed anger when they sinned.

Recognize there is a massive difference between God's anger and the anger we typically show. God is "slow to anger" (Ex. 34:6). Anger is not His first reaction to us nor is it His last. J. I. Packer says, "God's wrath in the Bible is never the capricious, self-indulgent, irritable, morally ignoble thing that human anger so often is. It is, instead, a right and necessary reaction to objective moral evil. God is only angry where anger is called for."[1] Packer believes "God's wrath ... is always judicial—that is, it is the wrath of the Judge, administering justice. Cruelty is always immoral, but the explicit presupposition of all that we find in the Bible ... is that each receives precisely what he deserves."[2]

God's wrath toward individuals or nations is directly related to their actions and choices. Before hell is an experience inflicted by God, it is a state humankind chooses. The last judgment upon the lost is the judgment they pass upon themselves by rejecting the light that comes through Jesus Christ. It is clear that God feels anger; yet His wrath is righteous, whereas ours most often is self-serving.[3]

Read Mark 11:15-17. How would you characterize the anger Jesus felt in this situation? (circle all that apply.)

deserved   immature   righteous   overdone

destructive   holy   purposeful

How is Jesus' anger in this situation like/unlike your most frequent expressions of anger?

_____

Jealousy

"Me jealous? You have got to be kidding," said Tom. "I'm not jealous! I'm just concerned." With that he turned and walked away from his frustrated girlfriend. Tom obviously was jealous but unwilling to admit it. Jealousy is a potent emotion that has held many lovers in its powerful grasp. It can lead to horrible acts of violence. What an explosive emotion!

"On reaching Jerusalem, Jesus entered the temple area and began driving out those who were buying and selling there. He overturned the tables of the money changers and the benches of those selling doves, and would not allow anyone to carry merchandise through the temple courts. And as he taught them, he said, 'Is it not written:

" 'My house will be called a house of prayer for all nations'?

But you have made it 'a den of robbers.' "
—Mark 11:15-17

What do you think of this statement: God gets jealous. My first reaction is to think it seems a little beneath God to become jealous. It is difficult to picture God loving us so much that when we are attracted to less-satisfying lovers, He would respond with jealousy. But that is exactly what the Bible says.

Look at Exodus 20:4-5: "You shall not make for yourself an idol. ... You shall not bow down to them or worship them; for I, the Lord your God, am a jealous God." A passage that helps us understand God's jealousy is Isaiah 54:5, "Your Maker is your husband." Our relationship with God is so intimate that the most accurate way to express it is to compare it to the relationship of a husband and wife.

What a mystery! God cares for us like a lover. Now let me assure you that God's jealousy is much different than the raw, carnal, human sort. It is righteous because it seeks our best. If God were to allow us to be attracted to anyone besides Himself, it would leave us unfulfilled, empty, and hopeless. He is the only One who will ever satisfy our hearts. A counterpart to God's jealousy is His love.

> "Do not worship any other god, for the Lord, whose name is Jealous, is a jealous God."
> —Exodus 34:14

 After you read this statement, circle the words that reflect your feelings: God is jealous of your affections, and He wants an intimate relationship with you.

happy   puzzled   honored   surprised   put off

humbled   eager   hesitant   afraid

Unconditional Love

That cold night on the Titanic when all knew that death was certain for many on board, numbers of men stepped aside so the children and women could get into the lifeboats. Their love was expressed by self-sacrifice. Such a scene stirs the depths of the human heart. We are forever changed.

Sacrificial love is perhaps the first emotional characteristic of God we are taught: "God so loved the world that he gave his one and only Son" (John 3:16). Of all the emotions of God, love is the only one used to define His essence. First John 4:7-8 paints this beautiful picture of God: "Dear friends, let us love one another, for love comes from God. Everyone who loves has been born of God and knows God. Whoever does not love does not know God, because God is love."

These verses give us a glimpse into the very heart of God. If we could open up His heart and look inside, we would find love as the foundation of His Being. With love as the core of His being, we must understand that all of His behaviors are motivated by love. That is great news! Our God and Savior has one motive in His heart toward us and that is love. God is love! Love is the axis on which all the other emotions of God revolve.

UPREACH

Praising God is one of the best ways we show our love for Him. Read a psalm of praise such as Psalm 96. Say it to God as you read.

 Do you believe God loves you? How has he shown His love? Thank Him for one or more of those ways right now.

Caring Compassion

In Exodus 34:6 God describes Himself. The first characteristic He names is *compassion*. Compassion compelled Him on numerous occasions to rescue His wayward people from a wicked enemy. The Book of Judges recounts God's intervention to save Israel from outside invaders. He preserved His sinful nation despite the fact that they had been unfaithful to Him. In other words, He showed compassion. Judges 10:16 records, "He could bear Israel's misery no longer."

Like His Father, Jesus is compassionate. Jesus went into the cities and villages around Him preaching, teaching, and healing. Matthew said, "When he saw the crowds, he had compassion on them, because they were harassed and helpless, like sheep without a shepherd." The word *compassion* could be translated *pity*. If you want to know how the heart of God responds to people's needs, go no further than this passage. The people were without direction, wandering like lost sheep. How did God respond? He sent His Shepherd Son to die for the sheep.

One need only thumb through the pages of the Gospels to see Jesus' compassion continually expressed as He healed the sick and restored those burdened with sin.

Read Matthew 15:32 in the margin. Why did Jesus feel compassion for the people? (Check one.)
❏ They had been listening to a long sermon.
❏ Not everyone was healed.
❏ They had nothing to eat.

The emotional expressions of God that I have named do not begin to comprise a complete list. We could talk about God's kindness or patience, for example. Do you find it interesting that He permitted the writers of the Bible to record for all time both His dark and bright emotions? God could have struck from the record any reference to anger or sadness, but He chose to leave it for us to read today. Can we conclude that anger and sadness are acceptable parts of our personhood?

God is far from being an impersonal, impassive figure disassociated from the universe He created. If God had not been an emotional Being, why would He have cared to create us at all? God's emotional nature is a significant key to understanding why we have emotions and what role they play in God's design.

WHY ARE WE EMOTIONAL?

Reread the Verse to Know for this week on page 15. Scholars have debated the implications of our being made in the image of God. Certainly we do not believe that God has a body identical to ours or that He is limited by time, space, or knowledge. God is omnipotent (all powerful), omnipresent (everywhere at once), and omniscient (all knowing). If being made in God's image does not give us unlimited intellect or freedom from physical limitations, what does the phrase mean? Some interpret it to mean that we are spiritual beings, that is, capable of relating to Someone outside of our earthly realm. Included in our spiritual nature is the ability to experience and express emotions. We are commanded to love our

"Jesus called his disciples to him and said, 'I have compassion for these people; they have already been with me three days and have nothing to eat. I do not want to send them away hungry, or they may collapse on the way.' "
—Matthew 15:32

Creator, each other, and ourselves (see Mark 12:30-31). An essential part of being like God is emotional expression.

Human Emotions

God has a rich and bountiful emotional landscape. Humans are like God in their emotional make-up. The Bible portrays men's and women's emotions as vividly as their Maker's. They displayed both bright and dark emotions, just as we do.

Bright Emotions

You can see it in the broad smiles of parents whose child is graduating from college after four years of hard work. It can be seen on the face of a grandparent holding a new grandbaby for the first time. A young man's face will beam with this emotion when he hears the woman he loves accept his marriage proposal. These are just a few of the faces of joy.

Joy has a strong physical component. For instance, when young children are joyful, their bodies tell you so. They might jump up and down, run excitedly around the room, or sing happy songs loudly. Adults, on the other hand, have learned to control their emotions (and this may not always be good!) so it is more difficult to know just how much joy they are experiencing. Here are some indications of adult joy. People may have bright, twinkling eyes as you look into them. It is as if the eyes are saying, "Isn't this great!" Broad smiles may cover their faces; the whole face radiates delight. Another clue is happy fidgetiness. They seem unable to stand or sit still for long. Look closely at my attempts to describe joy. Did you notice anything particular about the descriptions? Joy is most often communicated without words. A person's body shows you joy long before it is spoken.

In Genesis 2 Adam is ecstatic. Why? God has just brought to him a companion like himself. Not a zebra, a hawk, or a crocodile, but a woman, his companion for life! These words rang forth from his heart, "This is now bone of my bones and flesh of my flesh; she shall be called 'woman,' for she was taken out of man" (Gen. 2:23). Adam was one joyful fellow.

When God drowned the Egyptians in the Red Sea, Moses sang a song of triumph to God (see Ex. 15). Miriam and other women took musical instruments and danced before the Lord. Spoken words were inadequate to express the joy in their hearts, so they sang and danced instead.

Acts 3 records Peter and John passing a beggar as they walked to the temple to pray. In the name of Jesus Christ, Peter healed him. Although he had been lame from birth (Acts 3:2), the man stood for the first time. What a sight! Then he walked, leaped, and praised God (v. 8). Now that is joy!

Another bright emotion is peace. I was overlooking the beach in South Carolina. The wind blew strongly over the turbulent and agitated waters. They crashed continually against the sandy shore. It seemed that the ocean was restless and nervous. I left the beach and returned in a couple of hours. I was not prepared for the

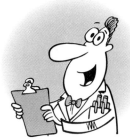

Professor Phitt says:
Recall from week 1 that your food choices can affect your mood. A sugary dessert may feel good at the time but a couple of hours later, the blood sugar level in your body dips, leaving you feeling down. Today choose foods that will elevate your mood naturally—not artificially— such as fruit and grains.

change in the ocean. The wind had ceased; the waves were calm. That calmness is a wonderful picture of peace. Peace has neither waves of worry nor strong winds of anxiety. We feel restful, not restless. All is well!

Peace is a state of relaxation. When I am peaceful, I no longer need to scan the environment for threat or danger. I am safe within the fold of the Good Shepherd. The assurance of His love and protection saturate my being. Let me give you an example. A mother and her six-year-old daughter are on a small prop-driven plane when it hits stormy weather. The ride is quite turbulent; many of the adult passengers are visibly shaken. But when we look at the small child, we see an unusual sight. She is lying across her seat with her head in her mother's lap—asleep. What a contrast to the adult passengers. She is at peace because she is close to her mom. That is the peace that God intends for us to have because of our closeness to Him.

 We can only scratch the surface of human emotions in one study. There are many other bright emotions. At what times are you most likely to feel and express bright emotions?

_____

_____

Dark Emotions

Dark emotions are those we associate with negative feelings. They convey the idea of being in a dark room isolated from others.

Even a strong, mature leader such as Moses could be doused with discouragement and despair. The children of Israel were complaining because they had no meat (see Num. 11). God had provided manna, yet they wanted something else (sounds like me). Verse 10 says the people were weeping at the door of Moses' tent.

The weight of their complaints became so heavy that Moses asked God, "Why have You afflicted Your servant? And why have I not found favor in Your sight, that You have laid the burden of all these people on me? Did I conceive all these people? Did I beget them, that You should say to me, 'Carry them in your bosom, as a guardian carries a nursing child,' to the land which You swore to their fathers? Where am I to get meat to give to all these people? For they weep all over me, saying, 'Give us meat, that we may eat.' I am not able to bear all these people alone, because the burden is too heavy for me. If You treat me like this, please kill me here and now—if I have found favor in Your sight—and do not let me see my wretchedness!" (v. 11-15, NKJV). Moses was so discouraged he wanted to die.

Like Moses, another great biblical hero of faith wanted to die from discouragement. Having seen God provide a marvelous victory over the prophets of Baal did not comfort Elijah when Jezebel threatened his life. First Kings 19:3 (NKJV) says he "ran for his life." In exhaustion he sat down under a tree in the wilderness. In utter despair and despondency he cried to God to take his life. "It is enough! Now,

OUTREACH

Last week you were asked to think about how your emotions affect those around you. This week ask, *How do others' emotions affect me?* Both dark and bright emotions are contagious. Watch which ones you "catch."

Lord, take my life, for I am no better than my fathers!" (v. 4, NKJV). Elijah's darkness was so great and his failure so devastating that death was the only solution he could see at the time.

We tend to think of biblical heroes as unlike ourselves; yet when we read their accounts, we find many of the same fears, anxieties, misgivings, and doubts that plague us. However, we also find ourselves identifying with their joy, pleasure, love, and gratitude.

You may ask, *so what?* How does finding biblical examples of the wide range of emotions affect my emotional wellness?

 Read again the subtitle of this study—the words after the title. Write them in the space below.

_____

We are seeking to follow the Creator's design. His plan will lead us to emotional wellness—wellness that is expressed emotionally in ways that please and honor Him. If you are willing, pray this prayer with me or say one of your own.

> *Dear God, thank You for making me in Your image. Thank You for being an emotional God and for sharing Your emotional Self with me. Thank You that I can feel all of my feelings—even the dark ones—with Your approval. Help me through this study and all You are doing in my life to learn to express my emotions in ways that build relationships with You, with others, and with myself. Amen.*

Our Purpose

Because we are God's children, we reflect the character and nature of our Creator. Often, our emotions are internal. We may think we are not revealing them to others, but our emotions are usually evident to others through our behavior. We really cannot hide the fact that we are emotional beings.

Our purpose in this study involves more than recognizing and valuing our emotional expression. This study is designed to help you grow in emotional wellness so that your emotional expression builds relationships and glorifies your Creator.

Think about the coming weeks. Set some goals for what you hope to learn, habits you wish to change, and new behaviors you want to incorporate into your life. Consider setting goals that also reflect your desire for good nutrition and adequate exercise. Use the information from pages 14-23 in your *Accountability Journal* make informed choices. Refer to these goals throughout the coming weeks to track your progress. Our *Fit 4* motto states, Wellness is achieved one step at a time.

The Creator's plan will lead us to emotional wellness.

This study is designed to help you grow in emotional wellness so that your emotional expression builds relationships and glorifies your Creator.

Fill in the information below to express your goals for this study.

I hope to learn:

_____

_____

_____

I wish to change these emotional habits:

_____

_____

_____

I want these new behaviors to characterize my emotional expression:

_____

_____

_____

I want to achieve these additional wellness goals:

_____

_____

_____

_____

_____

[1] J. I. Packer, *Knowing God* (Downers Grove: InterVarsity Press, 1973), 136.
[2] Ibid., 137.
[3] Ibid., 138.

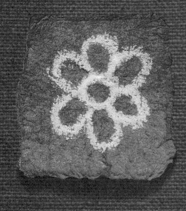

Examining Your Emotional History

This week you will look at some of the main factors that have contributed to your emotional development. View them as the foundation of your emotional self. Seek to understand the role each has played so that you can continue your lifelong journey to maturity. Don't feel singled out by this list. These factors influence all of us: our sin nature, our culture, trauma, the church, our families, and temperament and personality.

OUR SIN NATURE

In the beginning God created Adam and Eve emotionally, spiritually, mentally, and physically healthy. God provided for them a beautiful garden, a spouse, a job (including a great retirement plan), and friendship with Himself. Their relationship with the Creator was characterized by a rich, deep, emotional intimacy; as a result, they experienced emotional intimacy with each other as well. It is impossible to achieve emotional wellness, or any other aspect of wellness, apart from intimacy with God. Adam and Eve knew a security, acceptance, and purpose that we only partially experience because of sin's entrance into our world.

 Before the fall there was no sin or disconnection from God. Write what it would have been like emotionally for Adam and Eve in the garden.

_____

_____

An Emotional Paradise

We read these words in Genesis 2:25 (NLT): "Now, although Adam and his wife were both naked, neither of them felt any shame." Shame is a feeling that something is inherently wrong with me; I didn't do something wrong—I am wrong. Imagine a life with no form of shame. God's presence and provision were so rich and satisfying that the man and woman were totally comfortable with God and with each other. This emotional paradise was soon to change.

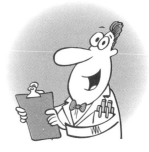

Professor Phitt says:
Read Genesis 1:29. The *Fit4* Guidelines for Healthy Eating (see page 20 in the *Accountability Journal*) remind us of the importance of eating 3 to 4 servings of fruit and vegetables each day.

Paradise Lost

Adam and Eve turned away from God and to themselves as they ate the forbidden fruit (Gen. 3:6). The taking of the fruit reflected the couple's distrust of God's goodness, although He had never failed them. Trusting themselves rather than God resulted in a cataclysmic change for the couple and the rest of humanity. Every aspect of Adam and Eve's life (spiritual, mental, physical, relational, and emotional) was forever distorted because of this act. Genesis 3:10 describes the beginning of emotional pain. Read Adam's words in the margin.

"I heard you in the garden, and I was afraid because I was naked; so I hid."
—Genesis 3:10

 Did you catch the emotional word in Adam's response? Write it here:

_____

The cold clasp of fear was a new feeling, one that had never before surrounded the fragile heart of man. For the first time, he fled from the One who had been closer to him "than a brother" (Prov. 18:24). How emotionally traumatic this must have been for Adam! All he had known was emotional bliss, yet now he lived in a shattered world inhabited by dark emotions. The emotional terrain of his and Eve's lives would never be the same. Never.

Cain, Adam's oldest son, experienced a different dark emotion. Genesis 4:5 (NLT) says, "This made Cain very angry and dejected." Cain's anger culminated in the murder of his brother, Abel. Humankind did not gradually become wicked sinners. It happened instantly and automatically progressed generationally.

The Impact of the Fall

In our culture, *sin* is not a politically correct word. In fact, many intellectuals and elitists deny the concept of sin. They talk about human mistakes, failures, improper actions, and wrong choices as though evil does not exist. Acts of abuse or violence are blamed on environment, poverty, lack of education, and past experiences.

"Put to death, therefore, whatever belongs to your earthly nature: sexual immorality, impurity, lust, evil desires and greed, which is idolatry."
—Colossians 3:5

The reason for their rejection of sin is obvious. The presence of sin requires a Savior. No one but God can forgive sins. Sin implies a heart that needs a makeover—a transformation rather than a cosmetic fix. The Bible refers to it as *a new nature.*

 Read Colossians 3:5 in the margin. Underline the characteristics of the old sin nature we inherit by birth.

"The sinful nature desires what is contrary to the Spirit, and the Spirit what is contrary to the sinful nature. They are in conflict with each other, so that you do not do what you want."
—Galatians 5:17

The human dilemma outlined by Paul in Galatians 5:17 is simply too true to be funny: My sinful nature fights for control with my spiritual nature so that I don't do what I know is right. No one born since Adam and Eve has been untouched by the scourge of emotional pain that started with a simple act of distrust in God.

 This week you are to examine your emotional heritage. Do you believe that you are a sinner by birth, separated from a holy God? ❑ Yes ❑ No Have you accepted Jesus Christ's sacrifice on the cross as payment for your sin? ❑ Yes ❑ No

If you have not made the decision to allow Jesus to be the Savior and Lord of your life, turn to page 87 and read how to become a Christian. If you have accepted Jesus as Savior, your relationship with God has been restored. You still have a sin nature, but your new nature gives you the power to resist temptation when you call on the Holy Spirit. Read 1 Corinthians 10:13 in the margin.

I wish that becoming a Christian settled the sin issue. Unfortunately, saved persons continue to sin. The differences between the saved and unsaved are significant, however.

1. The saved do not pay the ultimate price for their sins. Jesus paid the price.
2. The saved do not continue in known sin. (The key word is *known*. If the Holy Spirit is convicting you of a particular sin, pay close attention. He won't give up, so you might as well let it go.)
3. Saved persons experience remorse for their sins. This remorse—the work of the Holy Spirit—leads to repentance (a turnaround—going the opposite direction from the way you were headed). Repentance leads to confession, and confession leads to God's forgiveness.

 Can you think of a specific sin that has cost you dearly in terms of emotional wellness? In the margin, write a prayer of thanks for God's forgiveness and for the new start He offers each of us every day.

OUR CULTURE

In addition to our sin nature, a second major influence on our emotional wellness is the culture in which we were nurtured. Some cultures are more family-centered, with an emphasis on community. Others are very individualized, with personal rights ahead of community concerns. Others diminish the individual and elevate the government's status.

Each morning my first-grade class stood together facing the flag, placed our small hands over our hearts, and said the Pledge of Allegiance. This experience taught me to appreciate a nation "under God," with individual freedom and a court system that protects the rights of the individual. Alongside these virtues, I learned some things as a part of my culture that I believe can stunt emotional maturity.

We Prize the Intellect

Our nation is known for its great thinkers and inventors—the Wright brothers, Thomas Edison, Alexander Graham Bell, and Henry Ford, to mention a few. Education is available to all. Many in our culture believe training the mind is the ultimate goal of life. Being a lifelong learner and developing your intellect are worthy pursuits. The danger comes when it is all you pursue. Thinking is one part of our personhood. Over-emphasizing any one part can lead to imbalanced living.

Can you imagine a world where everyone resembles Spock on Star Trek? To him and his race the mind was everything. He could neither feel emotions nor recognize them in others. Maintaining balance between mental and emotional development

"No temptation has seized you except what is common to man. And God is faithful; he will not let you be tempted beyond what you can bear. But when you are tempted, he will also provide a way out so that you can stand up under it."
—1 Corinthians 10:13

"If we confess our sins, he is faithful and just and will forgive us our sins and purify us from all unrighteousness."
—1 John 1:9

My Prayer:

will help us be all God created us to be. Dallas Willard believes, "Being a man of the scriptures, Jesus understood that it is the care of the … whole person, that must be our objective if we are to function as God designed us to function."[1]

We Deify Achievement

We are the nation that offers the opportunity to make a million dollars even if you start with very little financially. We say, "Just set your mind to it! If you work long enough and hard enough, you can accomplish anything." Americans are "doers" at heart. Listen to the conversations around you that illustrate our performance mentality. We will tell you about our jobs, degrees, hobbies, clubs, civic organizations, ball teams, and so forth. We clearly believe we are what we do! We do not know how to rest, relax, and replenish.

We Devalue Relationships

The pursuit of intellect and achievement allows very little room for relational development. In fact, it can squeeze the life out of relational intimacy. A person can be recognized as brilliant intellectually or as a gold medalist in achievement and have little to no relational competence. What a tragedy! It is not difficult to understand why family breakdown is a major problem or why the divorce rate remains high. What is one to conclude about the impact of our culture on emotional development?

1. Emotions are minimized. To the intellectual, emotions do not fit in nice, clear-cut categories. The achiever dislikes emotions because they slow down the next accomplishment.
2. The language of emotions is spoken by few people. Linguists often study "dead" languages. In some ways emotional language is a dying, if not dead language. The journey to emotional wellness is not a crowded six-lane interstate. It is more like a deserted, overgrown trail leading through the forest. We must look closely to see the signs of those who traveled before us.
3. We must have a higher goal than others' approval if we are to successfully reach our goal: knowing Christ in all aspects of our being, not just in our minds and behavior. Recall the words of the prophet Jeremiah in our Verse to Know for this week (p. 25). The whole heart consists of soul, mind, strength, and emotions. Ask God for His guidance as you intentionally pursue emotional wellness.

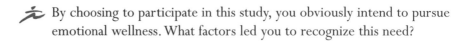 By choosing to participate in this study, you obviously intend to pursue emotional wellness. What factors led you to recognize this need?

_____

_____

THE ROLE OF TRAUMA

Have you ever watched a potter work? I was amazed at how the potter's hands could take a rough slab of red clay, throw it onto the wheel, and fashion it with his

> The pursuit of intellect and achievement allows very little room for relational development. In fact, it can squeeze the life out of relational intimacy.

hands into a beautiful vase. Once his work was done, the piece was fired in a kiln and sold. Trauma is like a potter; people are similar to clay. Painful and disruptive circumstances, like massive hands, can leave deep, lasting impressions on us emotionally. Let's look at different types of trauma that impact emotional wellness.

War

"I just can't get Vietnam out of my mind," Jack said. He was slumped over in his chair as if unable to bear the pain any longer. The pastor listened as Jack told how he woke up in a cold sweat at night from terrifying flashbacks. At work he could hear a particular sound or smell a specific scent that immediately transported him back to the rice paddies of Viet Nam. War overloads and short-circuits the emotional system. One way to handle the pain is denial. Many veterans simply try to block out their gut-wrenching emotions.

Disaster

Even though Julie is 35, she still remembers the day the twister demolished her home. She was six at the time. Her mom rushed into the house, scooped her up frantically, and headed to the bathroom at the center of the house. Julie could see the fear on her mom's face as they sat facing each other in the bathtub. Then it happened! The wind sounded like a mighty train engine as it ripped through their house. She remembers the house shaking and wood flying everywhere. Her last memory was of being picked up and tossed like a rag doll. She and her mom were thrown 20 yards from their home. Both of them survived, even though they had lengthy hospital stays. The trauma is not over for Julie. Whenever the skies get dark or strong winds blow, she is still gripped with fear.

Abuse

Survivors find abuse most difficult to talk about because of the deep shame associated with it, yet abuse is a major cause of emotional pain. Abuse takes on many forms: physical, sexual, emotional, verbal, and spiritual. The number of people in our country who have been touched by abuse is staggering. We are told that one in three girls and one in five boys will be sexually abused by the time they are 18. Abuse of any sort can be emotionally crippling. A child who is sexually abused will experience tremendous emotional extremes. He or she can be peaceful one minute, then suddenly be plunged into the depths of anxiety or fear.

Those Who Observed Abuse

"What is wrong with me?" Tom asked his friend Jim. "I understand why my sister is depressed and anxious, because she was sexually abused by Dad. But why do I live with so much emotional pain? He never did a thing to me!" Tom is one of a growing number of people who experience secondary trauma from having observed someone being abused or having been physically near a victim. The abuse observer is traumatized similarly to the abuse victim. The number of those emotionally impacted by abuse is multiplied.

The traumas we have mentioned are not a complete list, but they give us examples of how painful events shape and impact our emotions.

OUTREACH
You may care deeply for someone who has been victimized by trauma. Your emotional involvement will produce good fruit if you take the time to learn more about the effects of trauma and how caregivers can best respond. In the appendix of both basic *Fit4* courses, *Nutrition* and *Fitness*, you will find a list of resources to help you be a more effective caregiver.

Have you experienced any of these types of trauma? ❑ Yes ❑ No
Have you experienced a trauma we have not listed? ❑ Yes ❑ No
How has trauma impacted your emotions? In the margin, write a sentence, phrase, or simply list words that come to your mind.

THE CHURCH

Church experiences can broaden and deepen our emotional lives, as we sing, pray, praise, and confess. William Kirwan says, "Regrettably … emotions have been unjustifiably de-emphasized in the evangelical church."[2] Why has this happened?

If you were to look at the history of the church, you would see cycles of the church impacting the world and cycles of the world impacting the church. In my opinion, some of the church's bias against emotions is the result of the culture we live in. The body of Christ is simply reflecting the world's belief system.

Some Leaders Teach Emotions Are Bad

"It does not matter what you feel," the pastor said in a booming voice. "Those feelings can lead you astray. Faith has nothing to do with feelings. Simply put your trust in Christ." This Christian leader viewed emotions as the archenemy of the faith. To him they should be rejected—all the time at all cost.

 Can you recall a similar statement made by a Christian leader or church member? Write it in the margin. Include your reaction to the leader's statement.

Transparency and Authenticity Are Often Ignored

Rather than encouraging openness and vulnerability, church members are often more comfortable with the pretense of health. Check this out—try saying how you really feel in your Bible study class or in a prayer meeting and see what happens. You may get shocked or disdainful looks from the group. Perhaps we ignore transparency and authenticity in order to avoid people's emotional messes. Yet, spiritual growth is nurtured by honesty. We need truth in the inward parts (Ps. 51). I encourage you to practice honesty in your church relationships.

"A broken and contrite heart, O God, you will not despise."
—Psalm 51:17

 What is your comfort level with openness? Check all that apply.
❑ I prefer being authentic and transparent.
❑ I don't mind if others are authentic and transparent.
❑ I rarely feel comfortable sharing my inner self.
❑ I would prefer others keep their thoughts and feelings to themselves.

Emotional Expression Becomes Emotionalism

Some churches swing to the other extreme of emotionalism, where major decisions and staffing are based on who sheds the most tears or seems the most fervent—not who presents the most logical case. Being overly emotional is as unbalanced as suppressing emotions.

Can you think of a situation in a church you've attended in which emotions ruled and a well-thought-out proposal got squelched? Write about it in the margin.

The goal of this study is to challenge you to seek God's help in developing emotional health since there are so few guides. As you encounter emotionally well individuals in your church, seek to learn from them. Encourage them in their journey toward open and honest emotional expression.

YOUR FAMILY

Each of us bears an emotional fingerprint from the family in which we were reared. Early on we were blank emotional canvases on which our parents painted their meaning of life. Then, somewhere along the way, we caught a glimpse of another family's canvas—one quite different from the one drawn by our family. It was strange at first, but we were at least curious. The shapes and designs were mesmerizing because we had never seen such bright or such dark colors. We had just been introduced to a family who lived differently from anything we had known.

 Reproduce the canvas you grew up with. What emotions were most commonly expressed? Place a check by who expressed them.

EMOTION	FATHER	MOTHER	OTHER
_____	❏	❏	❏
_____	❏	❏	❏
_____	❏	❏	❏
_____	❏	❏	❏

Certain emotions may have been directly encouraged and reinforced by a parent. "Oh, look at that smile! What a happy baby!" Other parents may have made statements like "Stop crying!" to halt emotional expression. Note that parents may be able to hinder the expression of an emotion, but they can never stop the experiencing of an emotion.

"Emotionless parents" seem to have no emotions. Their children grow up emotionally illiterate. Other parents give subtle, nonverbal cues that tell the child that emotional expression is unacceptable: a facial scowl, a squinting of the eyes, a shaking of the head, or a clearing of the voice. The child gets the message that those emotions are off limits.

 What emotions were off limits in your family? List them.

_____

UPREACH

The family you grew up
in was not an accident. God
allowed the circumstances of
your upbringing to mold you
into the person He wants
you to be. Whether or
not you understand
God's design for your life,
by faith thank Him for
your family of origin.

"All the days ordained for me
were written in your book
before one of them came
to be."
—Psalm 139:16

The other extreme is parents who over-experience every emotion. When they experience a strong emotion, it dominates their lives and the lives of those around them. A child with this type of parent learns to ignore his or her own feelings because the parent's emotions govern the family. This child may learn to over-identify with the feelings of others and never develop his own emotional center.

What would an emotionally healthy home look like? Here are some characteristics of those types of families.

1. A variety of emotions are permitted and encouraged. The family is comfortable with sadness, anger, frustration, joy, humor, and silence. The emotional tapestry of their lives is varied and diverse.
2. Extreme emotional expression is infrequent. This family would not see regular daily doses of raging, screaming, or sullen quietness. They know that unbridled emotional expression is dangerous and damaging.
3. The adults model effective listening when a family member is expressing emotions. They are able to be patient and less defensive.
4. These families laugh a lot. To be with them is to get the real sense that they enjoy each other. Fun is a regular part of their lives.

Which of the four characteristics were common in your home? Put a star beside them. Put an X beside those not characteristic of your family.

YOUR TEMPERAMENT AND PERSONALITY

Our sin nature, culture, trauma, church, and family all contribute to our emotional makeup. Now we turn our attention to how your temperament and personality contribute to emotional wellness. We know that no two people are emotionally the same. Dwight Carlson states that, "The data coming in, I believe, clearly show that emotionally we are not created equal."[3] I believe that is by the design of God. Psalm 139:13-16 tells us that God has a unique design for each person. You are one of a kind and that includes your experience and expression of emotions.

God chose to give you a particular temperament. By temperament I mean inborn traits or qualities. These traits are not something you develop or become. They are part of your uniqueness, what you were created to be by our Heavenly Father. To prove this point, just go to the maternity ward of any hospital and watch the group of cute little newborns. One is crying for all he is worth, another smiles, and yet another has very little response. They are expressing their temperament. For example, my son Chase was active, verbal, and independent from day one. My daughter Chelsea was quieter and more dependent. They came unique from birth. *Independence* or *dependence* is an example of temperament.

Another example of temperament is what has commonly been labeled *introversion* and *extroversion*. The extrovert is characterized by expressiveness, gregariousness, and social activity. The introvert needs less human interaction and prefers time alone in solitary activities. If you want to really frustrate yourself, try to get an introvert to be extroverted or vice-versa. It is impossible! These two styles are expressions of their true persons.

Using the following scales, rate yourself on these qualities by placing an X at the appropriate spot.

dependent   independent

introvert   extrovert

Do not attempt to change your temperament. A better idea would be to understand who you are, then adjust as necessary. For example, I believe I am an introvert, but I am able to function in an extroverted fashion for short periods. Unlike a true extrovert, I have to get away from the crowd and activity to replenish, or I begin to experience emotional warnings of exhaustion. Understanding—not changing—your temperament is the key!

Do you like and accept the person God created you to be? Perhaps you've been taught you are unacceptable in some ways. Begin today to tell yourself positive messages about the unique you. "Self-talk"—what we say to ourselves—can either hinder or help our emotional development.

Below are some examples of temperament types that are taken from *Leaving the Light On* by Gary Smalley and John Trent. Do you find yourself in one of these categories, or do you believe you are a mixture of two?

 Place a star beside the trait(s) most like you.

1. The Lion—strong, aggressive, take-charge types, doers, problems-solvers, decisive. They can have a take-no-captive mentality. They make fearless Marines, tough managers, and determined, visionary entrepreneurs. Meaningful conversation is not their strong suit. They live in the now!

2. The Otter—energetic, fun-loving, people-persons; excitable cheer-leaders; and motivators. They love to talk and give lots of input—the consummate networker. They communicate with much warmth. You are made to feel as if you are their best friend. They live in the future.

3. The Golden Retriever—loyal, supportive, nurturing encouragers. They have a difficult time saying no. They can absorb a great deal of relational bumps and bruises and yet stay committed. They are listeners and empathizers. They are a be-there-when-ya-need-me friend. They readily sense others' hurts. They live in the present.

4. The Beaver—gives much attention to detail, always wants to do things the right way, careful, methodic, and thorough to a fault. They read all instruction books front to back. They like maps, charts, and organization. They want precision and are willing to express bulldog persistence to get it.[4]

INREACH

Practice positive self-talk this week. Give yourself messages that build you up instead of tearing you down. What affirming word can you give yourself right now?

Now that you have identified at least one emotional temperament, what emotions do you think are common for your style? Make a list at the bottom of this page. Be prepared to discuss your list with your group.

YOUR STORY IS NOT FINISHED

We've been talking about your emotional history. History is in the past. That's a good word for us. No matter what your emotional history, those experiences do not have to characterize you in the present or future. Paul said we are a new creation, "the old has gone, the new has come!" (2 Cor. 5:17).

New opportunities to learn and grow. A transformed nature empowered by the Holy Spirit. A fresh start each day (see Lam. 3:22-23 in margin). Reread the Verse to Know (p. 25) and commit it to memory. God promises He will reveal Himself to those who genuinely seek Him. He holds the key to knowing who you were created to be. The degree to which your emotional past dictates your choices today is just that: your choice. Remember that wellness is achieved one wise choice at a time. During this study, practice wise emotional choices. We will deal with those choices and our responses in the coming weeks.

"Because of the Lord's great
    love we are not
    consumed,
  for his compassions never
    fail.
They are new every
    morning;
  great is your faithfulness."
—Lamentations 3:22-23

---

[1]Dallas Willard, *The Divine Conspiracy* (New York: HarperSanFranscisco, 1998), 352.
[2]William T. Kirwan, *Biblical Concepts for Christian Counseling* (Grand Rapids, MI: Baker Book House, 1984), 51.
[3]Dwight L. Carlson, M.D., *Why Do Christians Shoot Their Wounded?* (Downer's Grove, IL: InterVarsity Press, 1994), 52.
[4]Excerpted from LEAVING THE LIGHT ON ©1994 By Gary Smalley and John Trent PH.D. Used by permission of Multnomah Publishers Inc.

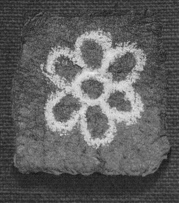

Week Four

Building Blocks of Emotional Wellness

Recall an experience in which you were aware of being effective. Perhaps you solved a problem, accomplished a task, or helped a friend. How did you feel about yourself at that moment? I would imagine you felt three particular feelings. These three feelings form the building blocks of emotional wellness. They undergird us when difficulties arise. What are they? Belonging, worth, and competence.

Dr. Maurice Wagner says, "These three feelings work together like legs of a tripod to support and stabilize self-concept. If any one of the three feelings is weak, the self-concept totters like a camera on a tripod when one leg is slipping. Each of these feelings is developed on a fundamental level in early childhood during the impressionable years. As one approaches adulthood and the state of responsible independence, he functions from this fundamental base of self-concept feelings."[1]

Dr. Wagner helps us understand the basic feelings necessary to develop emotional wellness from childhood to adulthood. Let's take a look at each of these three building blocks.

BELONGING

Belonging is the awareness of being wanted and accepted, of being cared for and enjoyed. It is a feeling that says confidently, "I fit with this group!" or "I am a part of this group!" Dr. Wagner believes a sense of belonging is established when loving parents anticipate their infants' discomforts and affectionately provide for their needs. This acceptance prepares them for better adjustment in future childhood years and for happier lives.[2]

 Think of a time between the ages of 6 and 10 when you particularly felt that you belonged. It could have been at home, school, church, or in another setting. Briefly identify the situation, and describe how you felt at that moment.

The opposite of belonging is sensing that you are on the outside looking in. Some family systems operate with an unwritten code that goes something like this: You are acceptable to this family as long as you_____ (fill in the blank). Belonging is held as a lure that can be snatched away as quickly as it is given. This transient sense of belonging leaves the family member always looking for acceptance—even in the wrong places.

 Every person experiences this sense of not belonging at some time. Think of a time in your adolescent years when you felt particularly left out. How did you feel at that moment?

_____

Often people who grow up in non-accepting family systems find it difficult to accept others. Having never felt they belonged, they may be unable to give others a sense of belonging. These individuals may develop a critical spirit toward others that results in fractured relationships. They may contribute to the same feelings of rejection in their children that they experienced from their own parents. A second possibility is that the individual will spend a lifetime trying to please and control others out of a sense of inadequacy. This lifestyle, often called codependency, is discussed in week 9 (see p. 78).

In a healthy family system, one's place in the family is never in doubt. Although a child may be disciplined for misdeeds or sense a parent's disappointment for specific actions, the child's inner sense of security and specialness survives these temporary bouts of feeling disapproval. Children need to have definite boundaries of acceptable conduct. However, at no time should the child sense a danger of losing his or her place in the family.

If you did not receive as much of a sense of belonging as you needed in childhood, we have wonderful news for you. Our marvelous Heavenly Father provides a true sense of acceptance and purpose despite the past and its deficiencies. When we look to Him for acceptance, He can provide what the world can never provide through wealth, beauty, popularity, or accomplishment. These worldly standards of belonging come and go. One minute you are a part of the "in crowd," and the next you are rejected, passé, old news.

How does God give us the only sure basis of belonging? When we accept Christ as our personal Savior and Lord, we become children of God.

"So you are no longer a slave, but a son; and since you are a son, God has made you also an heir."
—Galatians 4:7

 Read Galatians 4:7 in the margin. If you have experienced this new birth through Christ, underline the words from this passage that indicate your status in God's family.

If you have not experienced this new birth through Christ, turn to page 87 and read "How to Become a Christian."

I wish I could tell you that all problems with lack of self-acceptance and belonging disappear as soon as one becomes a Christian. However, God's change process may take a lifetime. At least in my case, a lifetime seems to be His timetable! I find comfort in Philippians 1:6. Read it in the margin.

You may wonder why I consider belonging to God's family so important. I am convinced that until we experience His unique gift of belonging, the other ways we find belonging will be fleeting and limited. No one—not your spouse, child, best friend, mentor, or boss—can make up the deficit you will invariably feel if you depend on something or someone else to give you personal security. Reread the Verse to Know for this week (p. 35).

"Being confident of this, that he who began a good work in you will carry it on to completion until the day of Christ Jesus." —Philippians 1:6

🏃 One aspect of belonging is spending time with the group to which you want to belong. Check the following activities that indicate your desire to experience a deep sense of belonging to God's family.
- ❏ spending time with God's family (regular worship with other believers, group Bible study, prayer group, fellowship, and social activities)
- ❏ contributing financially to the family's needs (tithing, special offerings)
- ❏ caring for the needs of the family (service through my church, volunteer opportunities)
- ❏ growing as an individual family member (personal prayer and Bible study, reading Christian books and magazines)

WORTH

Worth is a feeling of "I am good" or "I count" or "I am right," says Wagner.[3] Worth, like the feeling of belonging, is established in childhood as one relates to parents.

🏃 Unfortunately, we can learn to seek worth in all the wrong places. What are some ways you have seen people seek to build a sense of worth?

_____

_____

My wife Terri and I have had the privilege of bestowing a sense of worth on Chase and Chelsea, our two children. Years ago we noticed that we tended to attach worth to being successful at activities. Therefore, the kids could easily confuse their worth with successful performance. Terri and I quickly realized that we did not want our children to think worth is earned only by good behavior.

We knew that our Savior died for us when we were "dead in [our] transgressions and sins" (Eph. 2:1). Our relationship to Jesus is despite our unworthiness. We desired to communicate this type of worth to Chase and Chelsea by regularly saying to them, "We are so glad God gave you to us!" These words and others like them communicate that worth is not based solely on activity and performance. In the same way, your Heavenly Father is overjoyed that you have become His child. Your worth is based on His love for you, not what you accomplish for Him.

Your worth is based on His love for you, not what you accomplish for Him.

Read the account of Jesus' baptism in Matthew 3:13-17. What did God say about His Son? Fill in the blanks:

" 'This is my Son, whom I _____;

with him I am well _____' " (v. 17).

Notice that Jesus had yet to perform a miracle, walk on water, teach the multitudes, or rise from the dead. He had not begun His public ministry. God was pleased with Him without performance! Does this passage encourage you? It really blesses me!

Instead of worth, many biblical characters had feelings of worthlessness. The woman of Samaria Jesus encountered at the well (see John 4) felt unworthy to give Jesus a drink of water. Not only was she a Samaritan and a woman, but her reputation had been soiled because of her adultery. Jesus gave her the gift of worth: She went back to her village and faced those who had scorned her. " 'Come, see. ... Could this be the Christ?' " (v. 29).

What would it be like to be disloyal and unfaithful to someone to whom you had totally committed your life? Peter denied his Master and Savior not once but three times (Matt. 26:69-74), despite having promised to die with Him (v. 35). I can only imagine the anguish that must have gripped the heart of this disciple of the Lord Jesus. Only moments before, Peter had assured his Teacher that he would go to the death with Him—now he realized he had denied Jesus publicly three times. Verse 75 says he "wept bitterly."

Jesus restored Peter's sense of worth to the Kingdom when He encountered Peter on the seashore and gave him the responsibility of feeding His sheep (see John 21). The faithless one became the faithful shepherd of the church in Jerusalem.

Modern writers have popularized the idea that accepting one's own worth is essential to accepting the worth of others. Whether or not they realized it, Jesus was way ahead of them. Our *Fit 4* theme passage in Mark 12:31 says, " 'Love your neighbor as yourself.' " Jesus said, in effect, that if you cannot love yourself, you will find it difficult, if not impossible, to love others. INREACH is an essential component of mental wellness.

COMPETENCE

Wagner says competence is a feeling of adequacy, of courage, or hopefulness, of strength enough to carry out the tasks of daily life situations. It is the "I can" feeling of being able to face life and cope with its complexities.[4]

A gripping sense of inadequacy is common to many Bible characters. They were frequently overwhelmed with a sense of inferiority when faced with the task God gave them. Moses offers a good example. When God called him to be the human

INREACH
Do you agree that worth is not based solely on activity and performance? On what is it based? Be prepared to share your answer with your group.

38

instrument of deliverance for the children of Israel who had been in bondage to Egypt for many years, Moses responded to God's instructions by saying, " 'Who am I, that I should go to Pharaoh and bring the Israelites out of Egypt?' " (Ex. 3:11). Moses' "who am I?" statement is filled with self-doubt and inadequacy. As he did a quick self-inventory and surveyed the task God called him to do, Moses concluded that he was horribly insufficient. The rest of Exodus 3 and half of chapter 4 record Moses' attempt to convince God of his inferiority.

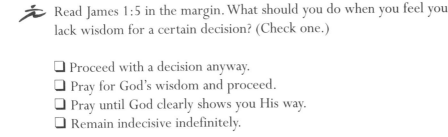 What circumstances bring out your feelings of inadequacy?

_____

_____

King David's son Solomon did not begin his reign with a lot of confidence. First Kings 3:7-8 records Solomon's sense of inadequacy. " 'I am only a little child and do not know how to carry out my duties. Your servant is here among the people you have chosen, a great people, too numerous to count or number.' " In essence Solomon told God that he was as helpless and weak as a little child who must be assisted to go in and out of his home. Solomon knew the task was impossible unless God was there, so he requested wisdom (1 Kings 3:9). When you experience inferiority or inadequacy, realize you are not alone. Ask for God's wisdom.

Read James 1:5 in the margin. What should you do when you feel you lack wisdom for a certain decision? (Check one.)

❑ Proceed with a decision anyway.
❑ Pray for God's wisdom and proceed.
❑ Pray until God clearly shows you His way.
❑ Remain indecisive indefinitely.

The biblical character Joseph is an example of someone who displayed a healthy sense of competence throughout his life. He faced one devastating problem after another, yet he always bounced back and became more successful. Joseph had to deal with the hatred of his brothers who sold him into slavery in a foreign land. In time, Joseph gained the respect of his Egyptian master, Potiphar, who made Joseph the overseer of all he possessed. Then when Joseph was unwilling to commit adultery with Potiphar's wife, she falsely accused him of trying to rape her, and he was put in prison. In prison he continued to demonstrate his competence. The prison official placed him in a position of leadership among his fellow prisoners. "The Lord was with Joseph and gave him success in whatever he did" (Gen. 39:23).

Joseph asked one of the prisoners he had helped to remember him when the man was released, but Joseph was forgotten for two years (Genesis 40:20—41:1). At the end of this two-year period, Joseph was summoned to Pharaoh's court. When he correctly interpreted Pharaoh's dream, Joseph was placed as second in command to Pharaoh. From that position he provided food for Egypt and his family.

"If any of you lacks wisdom, he should ask God, who gives generously to all without finding fault, and it will be given to him."
—James 1:5

UPREACH
In the following verse, underline our source of power for service to God.

" 'You will receive power when the Holy Spirit comes on you; and you will be my witnesses in Jerusalem, and in all Judea and Samaria, and to the ends of the earth.' "
—Acts 1:8

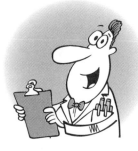

Professor Phitt says:
Our self-image tends to improve when we feel we are making wise choices. Use your *Accountability Journal* each day. Give yourself positive feedback about your exercise and nutrition choices. Perfection is not the goal. Wellness is achieved one wise choice at a time.

"I love you, O Lord,
    my strength.
The Lord is my rock, my
    fortress and my deliverer;
my God is my rock, in
    whom I take refuge.
He is my shield and the horn
    of my salvation, my
    stronghold."
            —Psalm 18:1-2

How did Joseph maintain competency in such difficult situations? "The Lord was with him." His competencies were based on a personal relationship with God, and Joseph made this abundantly clear to Pharaoh when Potiphar asked Joseph to interpret his dream. Joseph said, "I cannot do it, … but God will give Pharaoh the answer he desires" (Gen. 41:16). Joseph was sure that his ability to interpret dreams had very little to do with him—and everything to do with God.

Competence was the result of Joseph's intimacy with God, not his marvelous intellect or insight. It can be the same for us! We are competent not because of who we are but because of Whose we are. We belong to Jesus! His power fuels our lives. " 'In him we live and move and have our being' " (Acts 17:28).

 On a scale from 1-5, with 1 being low and 5 being high, rate the degree to which you feel a sense of belonging, worth, and competence. At your next group session, you will have the opportunity to share a time when you either experienced or lacked each of these three feelings.

belonging	1	2	3	4	5
worth	1	2	3	4	5
competence	1	2	3	4	5

You may feel you belong more in one situation than another; you may be more competent riding a bike than skiing downhill. What I am suggesting is that these three emotions must form the foundation of your self-concept before you will be likely to feel, express, and manage your emotions.

Our emotional expression has a way of indicating the absence of belonging (hurt feelings, feelings of abandonment, rejection), worth (inferiority, embarrassment, shame), and competence (inadequacy, failure syndrome, passivity). If you lack these foundational elements, remember that you must find these in relationship with your loving Heavenly Father. They cannot be granted by a spouse, friend, boss, or pastor. Our security must be firmly fixed in the only reliable source.

 Read Psalm 18:1-2 in the margin. Underline the words that reveal the source of David's security.

Pray this prayer with me or write your own in the margin.

> *Father, You know how I have struggled with belonging, worth, and competence. Thank You for showing me that I can't attain these through my own efforts. They are gifts from You as I claim my place in Your family. Teach me to look to You for belonging, worth, and competence. Amen.*

[1]Maurice E. Wagner, *The Sensation of Being Somebody* (Grand Rapids, MI: Pyranee Books, 1975), 32-33.
[2]Ibid., 34.
[3]Ibid.
[4]Ibid., 36.

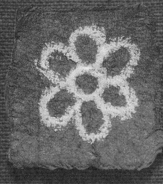

Week Five

Understanding Yourself and Others

The doctor checked my temperature and took my blood pressure. He said my lungs were clear of congestion and my heartbeat was normal. After peering into my eyes, ears, and nose, he concluded, "Physically, you are in good shape. Be sure to set an appointment for next year as you are leaving."

Wouldn't it be great if we could know we are emotionally healthy? A doctor can test for physical illnesses, but how does one test for sadness or unforgiveness? Emotions are not easily diagnosed, especially if we keep them hidden inside or deny them. Our Verses to Know remind us that our Creator knows us inside and out. He holds the key to understanding self and others.

This week we begin our study of the five components of emotional wellness suggested by Salovey and Mayer in Daniel Goleman's book *Emotional Intelligence*. The five are 1) understanding your emotions, 2) managing your emotions, 3) motivating yourself, 4) identifying emotions in others, and 5) developing relationships.[1]

Week 5 will examine the first and fourth components. In week 6 we will determine strategies for managing emotions. Week 7 will deal with using emotional energy as motivation for positive life changes, and week 8 will help us develop relationship skills, since emotions are the voice of relationships (see p. 12).

UNDERSTANDING YOUR EMOTIONS

Sue said, "I'm feeling discouraged today. This heaviness inside won't go away. I've felt it before but not quite this strong. Would you pray with me about this feeling?" Her husband Jim gently took her hand as they bowed their heads and prayed.

Sue has a good understanding of her emotions. She does not deny dark emotions when they show up. She pays attention without being overwhelmed or suffocated by them. She courageously attempts to tell God and others what is going on inside her. Jim, on the other hand, is confused and fearful about his emotions. Most of the time he is unsure what is going on inside emotionally. He is growing in his awareness, but unlikely to share his feelings with anyone.

How aware are you of your own emotions? (Check one.) Are you more like ❑ Jim? or ❑ Sue?

Why Don't I Understand My Emotions?

In week 2 we examined the emotions associated with God in the Bible. We, too, experience those emotions. However, our emotional expression has been corrupted by sin. As a result, our self-centered focus makes it very difficult for us to see ourselves objectively.

The fall (Genesis 3) produced a human heart that is easily deluded. Sin poses a monstrous barrier that makes knowing myself very limited—if not impossible. The best I can do apart from God is to get vague glimpses of myself. And I can never be sure that these glimpses are completely accurate. Only the Creator knows me inside and out. I must have a vital, growing, love relationship with God if I ever hope to understand myself. Not knowing what is going on inside of us should encourage us to go to God and ask Him to search our hearts. Reread the Verses to Know—Ps. 139:23-24—and commit them to memory. In this study, think of your heart as the real you. If all of the external scaffolding were stripped away, all that would be left would be the true you—the heart. That is what the psalmist asked the Lord to search.

 Ask God to search your heart. To what extent do you think you really understand yourself? (Circle one.)

almost entirely   a lot   some   little

What is Emotional Illiteracy?

The United States government has spent millions of dollars trying to stamp out reading illiteracy. My personal cause is to stamp out emotional illiteracy, especially for believers. To be emotionally literate, we need to identify and understand our emotions. Maybe you are one of many for whom this is a challenge. Perhaps you are unsure what people are talking about when they share feelings. To be emotionally illiterate is to be relationally handicapped. You cannot fully compensate with mind, spirit, or body. God intended full use of your emotions. What are some signs of emotional illiteracy? Here are some points to consider.

Emotionally Unaware

"Tom functions like a computer," said his wife Betty. "All he can do is think, analyze, and solve problems. Sometimes I wish he would just tell me what he is feeling inside. I am concerned because at times he seems totally disconnected from his emotional life. For instance, when his mom passed away, he did not shed a tear. As far as I know, he has never expressed any emotion over her loss. It seems odd because they appeared to be close. I'm not sure what to do or how to help him."

Tom is an example of someone who has very little emotional awareness or expression. He may not know that he has cut himself off from his emotions. He may even

---

"The heart is deceitful above all things and beyond cure. Who can understand it?"
—Jeremiah 17:9

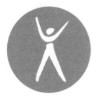

UPREACH
Emotional understanding can expand under the watchful eye of your Heavenly Father.
One result of God searching you is being able to recognize your emotions. Make Him an important part of your plan for increasing self-awareness.

believe there is nothing wrong with the way he is—that is, until he encounters a crisis or breaking point. Such a crisis may make him deal with his emotions. It may prompt him to work on emotional awareness by asking for God's help.

Bothered When Others Express Emotions

Joann will not allow her 10-year-old daughter, Megan, to cry when she hurts herself. She forcefully tells Megan, "Big girls don't cry. Stop it right now!" Megan tries to stop the tears. Usually it takes a while, which is even more irritating to Joann. It is not just Megan who irritates her, but anyone who is forthright with feelings or who expresses negative emotions. Joann believes you deal with feelings on the inside and go on. The quicker the better! Don't convey them openly.

Limited Feeling Vocabulary

Our vocabularies may be lacking when it comes to words that describe feelings. Jason's company was relocating him from Oklahoma to Oregon. His pastor asked Jason to describe his feelings about the move. Jason responded, "I wish you had asked me what I thought instead. I really do not know what I am feeling."

As the pastor helped Jason explore his feelings, it became apparent that he had a limited number of emotions he could identify clearly with words. Most of the time he responded to the pastor's inquiries with "I'm not sure." Eventually, Jason identified what was going on inside. As he understood himself better, he made decisions that reflected his new understanding. For example, to reflect his appreciation for nature, Jason chose to buy a house in a rural area rather than in the city.

 As you look at the characteristics of emotional illiteracy, do you identify with one or more of them? ❏ Yes ❏ No
How would becoming more emotionally literate affect your life?

_____

_____

Learning to recognize your emotions begins with naming them. As we have seen, naming your emotions requires expanding your feeling vocabulary.

 Look at the feelings chart on page 48. Study each picture and its word description. This week try expressing your feelings using words not commonly in your feeling vocabulary. Share the results with your group.

Continue to study the feelings chart over the next few weeks. Learning new feeling words will help you understand and express your emotions more accurately.

Historical Emotions

"Why was I so afraid?" Sam asked his friend Tim. "The feeling came out of nowhere! I just walked into the home where I grew up, and fear rolled over me like a massive wave. I was overwhelmed by it!"

INREACH

Identifying your emotions is the first step to managing them. Refer to the feelings chart on page 48 throughout this study. This chart will help you expand your feeling vocabulary.

A historical emotion is one that occurred earlier in life that is re-experienced later.

Sam's experience has the markings of a historical emotion—one that occurred earlier in life that is re-experienced later. The historical emotion has been repeatedly felt to the point that it takes up permanent residence in the individual. It lies dormant until a person experiences a series of events that reflect the earlier painful experience. At this point the emotion is reactivated and re-experienced.

1. Historical emotion can move you from feeling extremely calm to frantic in a matter of seconds, even milliseconds. Because you have experienced this emotion repeatedly, it seems to bypass the will and conscience.
2. Historical emotions leave you feeling perplexed. "Where did that come from?" or "What was that?" Trying to make sense out of the feeling from a present perspective will only be frustrating, because the key is in the past.
3. If you are unsure if an emotion has history, ask this question: "When and where have I felt like this before?" The answer will help you connect the present emotion to its origin.

Allow me to illustrate. Stan hated his father's domineering attitude. His dad had frequently shamed Stan in public. Stan believed he was free from these humiliating experiences until one day at work his boss "blew up." The boss's anger and harsh, condescending words overwhelmed Stan with a deep sense of shame and embarrassment. The boss had reactivated his old emotional pain—only Stan was experiencing it as an adult.

You will recall from week 3 that our emotions have a historical base. They originate in our families, churches, and culture, as well as being a part of our personalities, life experiences, and sin natures. If you discover that you commonly feel strong, dark, historical emotions, you may have significant past pain. Do not be afraid to seek professional help from a Christian counselor. Once you address these emotions, you will not be as easily overwhelmed or perplexed by them.

Sharing Your Emotions

Learning to recognize your emotions and to express them in appropriate ways is a vital part of God's design for emotional wellness.

Learning to recognize your emotions and to express them in appropriate ways is a vital part of God's design for emotional wellness. As you progress through this study, keep in mind the goal of self-understanding. As we understand ourselves, we can express ourselves to others more effectively. The most important information you have to communicate to a significant other is what you know about yourself.

Speak for Yourself

When you share emotional content with others, use "I" statements to convey your feelings. We often create defensiveness because our listeners hear us judging and blaming them with statements such as "You shouldn't do that" or "You never" or "You always." We can avoid a defensive reaction by being careful to speak only for ourselves, such as "I get really uncomfortable when I see you doing that."

Don't Make Assumptions

Often we mistakenly believe our listeners know exactly what we think, feel, and want. We may even say, "If he or she really loved me, my partner would just know." Others cannot climb into our skins or read our minds, regardless of how much they may care about us. We must be willing to communicate our feelings to them. Of course, the first step is self-awareness. Once we know what we think, feel, and want, it is our responsibility to communicate our wishes to others.

Focus on the Present

Little can be done about what has happened in the past. The most effective communication focuses on what is happening now. Perhaps past incidents have triggered your need to talk. However, the current situation should be the subject; the object should be to look for ways to resolve the issue for the future. Wrangling over who did or said something in the past rarely builds a relationship.

Keep It Simple

Simple statements about what is going on with you are preferable to a long introduction, many words, and an extensive summary. Overtalk can be just as damaging to a relationship as undertalk. Often our listeners tune us out or avoid us because they dread the long talk. After you share a concise statement, ask if your listener needs further clarification. If not, move on.

 Rate yourself on your ability to communicate your feelings with others, where 1 = needs improvement and 5 = I could lead a seminar on the subject. Circle one number beside each statement.

Speak for yourself.	1	2	3	4	5
Don't make assumptions.	1	2	3	4	5
Focus on the present.	1	2	3	4	5
Keep it simple.	1	2	3	4	5

UNDERSTANDING OTHERS

As Sara reflected on her conversation with Traci, she was amazed that Traci so easily identified with her feelings. Sara had struggled with obesity all of her adult life. Before meeting Traci she had concluded that no "thin" person could ever understand her dark struggle with food and self-hate. Her conversation with Traci caused her to re-think her opinion. Traci seemed to understand. Sara felt relieved that someone was able to hear her heart.

 Traci was able to identify with Sara. Do you recall a time when someone identified with the emotions you were experiencing? If so, tell about it.

_____

_____

If you thought of an example, you know that being understood is a wonderful blessing. Someone viewed life through your eyes. They did not judge or ignore you. Instead, they listened, heard your heart, and affirmed you.

"Praise be to the God and Father of our Lord Jesus Christ, the Father of compassion and the God of all comfort, who comforts us in all our troubles, so that we can comfort those in any trouble with the comfort we ourselves have received from God."
—2 Corinthians 1:3-4

"For this reason he [Jesus] had to be made like his brothers in every way, in order that he might become a merciful and faithful high priest in service to God, and that he might make atonement for the sins of the people. Because he himself suffered when he was tempted, he is able to help those who are being tempted."
—Hebrews 2:17-18

OUTREACH

Recall a time when you were able to identify with another person's emotions. Be prepared to share this experience with your group.

Empathy

The fourth characteristic of emotional wellness is the ability to identify emotions in others. Another word for this characteristic is *empathy*. *Webster's Ninth New Collegiate Dictionary* defines *empathy* as "the action of understanding, being aware of, being sensitive to, and vicariously experiencing the feelings, thoughts, and experience of another." A simpler definition is "the ability to hear and understand the heart of another."

Empathizing is becoming a lost art in our fast-paced culture. Empathy grows best in a non-hurried lifestyle, a lifestyle that can slow down enough to walk quietly and patiently with another. Jesus is our ultimate example of one who could empathize with others. Jesus experienced our feelings, thoughts, and life experiences. He became one of us. Read Hebrews 2:17-18 in the margin.

To empathize with others we must have inner security and stability that allow us to address others' needs. That is exactly what a relationship with Jesus does. It assures me that I am loved and provided for so adequately that I can turn my attention to others. Pray this prayer with me, or write one of your own in the margin.

Jesus, teach me to empathize as You do. You know how much time I spend focused on me and my needs. Thank You for the comfort I have received from You. Allow me to hear and understand the hearts of others. Amen.

Listening

The highest compliment you can pay another person is to listen to what he or she is saying. Listening is also the best way to understand that person. Listening is more than keeping quiet when someone else is talking. Often we simply use that time to rehearse what we will say next when the opportunity presents itself.

Active listening is a term often used to describe *effective listening*. Active listeners attempt to hear and understand the speaker's message. Note that I did not say the attempt to correct his thinking or to expound on what he has said. Listening is not about you but about others. Active listening ministers to them.

Examples of Ineffective Listening

1. The Fact Finder listens to find out who, what, when, where, and how. This type squelches emotional expression and puts the listener on the defensive.
2. Mr. Fix-it listens to solve the problem, and the sooner the better. A fix-it mentality depreciates the value of talking through problems and expressing feelings as important steps along the way to resolving issues.
3. Ms. Advisor is available if you want some advice. She is full of what you should have done or yet can do. By the way, don't bother to disagree with her solution. Her mind is made up. She also knows how you should feel about it.
4. The Judge listens intently, but he is full of guilt and recrimination. You are likely to leave this conversation feeling that you don't measure up to standard. You are certainly not likely to express your emotions.

5. The Robot appears to listen and nods at intervals, but it soon becomes apparent that the robot's mind is miles away. You may feel you were not worth his time and trouble, and you are not likely to share your feelings.

How do you feel when you encounter persons with these ineffective listening patterns? Check the words that apply.

❏ Diminished   ❏ Misunderstood   ❏ Sad   ❏ Angry

❏ Aggressive   ❏ Hostile   ❏ Frustrated   ❏ Discouraged

Effective Listening Skills

1. Create an environment for listening. Turn off the television or radio, put down the magazine or newspaper, and give the speaker your full attention.
2. Face the person and make eye contact. Lean forward. Use body language—a nod, a smile, a look of concern—to communicate that you are listening.
3. Do not interrupt. Wait for the speaker to complete his or her thoughts before expressing your own ideas. Do not appear to rush the speaker. Some people take a few seconds to collect their thoughts.
4. Use questions sparingly. When you do ask a question, consider asking an emotion-exploring one such as, "How did you feel about that?" Often how we feel is much more important than the cold facts of the situation.
5. Ask for clarification. Restating what you have heard helps to insure that you heard correctly. It also affirms the speaker. "He was really listening!"
6. Avoid biographical listening. This listener is quick to jump into the conversation with a similar story. "Wait until you hear what happened to me!" Biographical listeners communicate disinterest and disregard for the speaker.
7. Affirm the speaker. Say, "I appreciate your sharing that with me." Offer help, a prayer, or arrange another time to talk.

Place a check by the effective listening skills you want to implement.

Effective listening gives you important information about the speaker that will help you understand his or her thoughts, emotions, concerns, needs, hopes, and fears. Use this information wisely; never use the information to hurt the person or to break a confidence. Treat the conversation as privileged information.

If you can increase your ability to identify your emotions and the emotions of others, you have taken a major step toward emotional wellness. Increasing your emotional vocabulary will help you better understand yourself and others. Practicing empathy and honing your listening skills will improve your relationships.

Read again the Verses to Know on page 41. Remember that God sees you, knows you, and loves you completely. Find time today to praise Him, both for who you are right now and for who you are yet to become as you grow in Christlikeness.

---

[1]Daniel Goleman, *Emotional Intelligence* (New York: Bantam Books, 1995), 43.

"Everyone should be quick to listen, slow to speak and slow to become angry."
—James 1:19

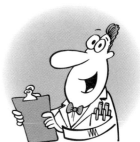

Professor Phitt says:
Understanding others begins with getting to know them. A good way to get to know other people is through exercise classes. Check with your church, gym, or other fitness facility about enrolling in an aerobics, step, kickboxing, stretching, water aerobics, or sports class. After class, meet for a nutritious drink or snack.

FEELINGS CHART

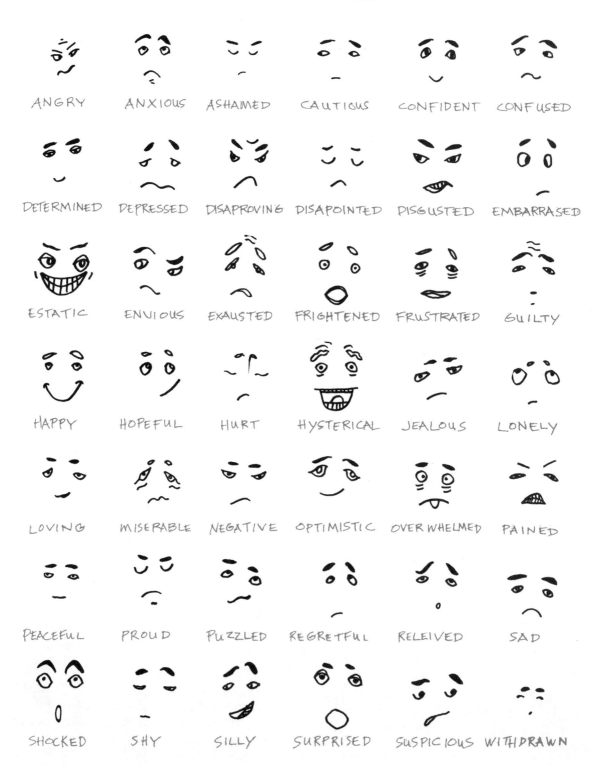

ANGRY ANXIOUS ASHAMED CAUTIOUS CONFIDENT CONFUSED

DETERMINED DEPRESSED DISAPROVING DISAPOINTED DISGUSTED EMBARRASED

ESTATIC ENVIOUS EXAUSTED FRIGHTENED FRUSTRATED GUILTY

HAPPY HOPEFUL HURT HYSTERICAL JEALOUS LONELY

LOVING MISERABLE NEGATIVE OPTIMISTIC OVERWHELMED PAINED

PEACEFUL PROUD PUZZLED REGRETFUL RELEIVED SAD

SHOCKED SHY SILLY SURPRISED SUSPICIOUS WITHDRAWN

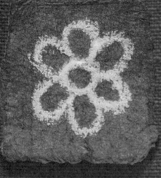

Managing Your Emotions

Bill was driving down the freeway when suddenly a red sports car cut directly in front of him, forcing him off the road and into the median. Fortunately, neither he nor his vehicle was hurt. But the same could not be said about his emotions. Once he brought his car to a complete stop, he slammed his fist into the steering wheel while shouting words of disgust and hatred toward the other driver. He threw his door open sharply, stepped out of the car, and forcefully kicked a soft-drink can lying in the grass. After a few minutes he came to himself and asked, "What is going on with me? All that rage and anger just came out of nowhere!"

Notice his words: "came out of nowhere!" For a few short minutes these invisible emotions seized control of his life.

 Can you relate to Bill's experience? Write a brief summary of a time when you were swept away by strong emotions that occurred in a short period of time, seemingly out of nowhere.

_____

_____

Managing emotions is not easy for anyone. We looked at the dark emotions of several biblical characters in week 2. Emotional wellness is more than identifying and feeling our feelings. This week we will look at five strategies for handling emotions in an appropriate way: avoid denial, practice self-control, practice solitude and stillness, journal thoughts and prayers, and look to God.

AVOID DENIAL

The mother walked into the kitchen, noticed her two-year-old son standing in front of the open refrigerator door, and called his name. When he turned around, she saw chocolate pudding smeared all over his face and on much of his little chest. He was doing his best to look innocent because he knew the pudding was off limits. Once the mother recovered from the initial shock, she decided to turn

"God did not give us a spirit of timidity, but a spirit of power, of love and of self-discipline."
—2 Timothy 1:7

49

this experience into a teaching time. She knelt down next to him and asked gently, "Did you eat the chocolate pudding, Aaron?" He vigorously shook his head no. She restated the question, "Aaron, Mommy wants to know if you ate the chocolate pudding in the refrigerator." Once again he shook his head and added, "No, Mommy. You told me I was not supposed to."

This story humorously illustrates denial. The little guy with pudding from head to chest said he had not been in the pudding at all. Even with a second try, the mom could not get him to change his view of reality. Who of us has not been in a similar circumstance? We use denial as a means of escaping painful reality. Denial is one way we cope with frustration, disappointment, loss, and pain. It serves as an emotional anesthetic, providing numbness and temporary relief. However, it distorts what is real, turning it into something less threatening and more bearable. Distorted reality does not change reality; it just changes our perception of it.

For example, a person in serious debt may make a substantial purchase and deny the reality of the new debt by saying, "I will cut back in other areas," or "A little more debt won't hurt." The denial may allow one to make the purchase, but it will be of no help when the bill comes. It only makes larger debt—that's reality. The Bible provides us with an illustration of denial's power in a believer's life. The story of David's adultery with Bathsheba is found in 2 Samuel 11—12.

 Read 2 Samuel 11:7-15. In the margin, explain how David tried to avoid the reality of his adultery. How does your answer compare with the following paragraphs?

David used varying forms of denial and distortion to cover his sin:
1. Deceptive Talk. As we listen to David's conversation with Uriah about the battle, his real concern was his need to cover up his adultery. All of his attention and energy was focused on hiding his sin. David's denial began with his words.
2. Manipulation. David attempted to manipulate Uriah into having sexual intercourse with his wife, Bathsheba, so it would appear that she was pregnant by her husband, not himself (v. 8-13). He tried to get Uriah drunk, thinking that when the man had less self-control, he would surely sleep with his wife. The king underestimated this leader's integrity and loyalty. Uriah would not sleep with his wife. The king's manipulation failed.
3. Destructive Actions. When manipulation did not work, David decided to have Uriah killed (11:14-27). In the process of having Uriah killed, others of David's army were killed as well (v. 17). In the end, David was flippant about the death of these men as is revealed in his message to Joab in verse 25, " 'Don't let this [the death of Uriah and others] upset you; the sword devours one as well as another. Press the attack against the city and destroy it.' " As David continued to deny and distort reality, he grew further and further away from God. He was so far from God that he was OK with what displeased God. What a frightening place to be! Denial damages our relationship to God.

"But the thing David had done displeased the Lord."
—2 Samuel 11:27

50

4. Disconnected from Self and God. Months had passed since David's original sin. Nathan the prophet brought a problem to the king having to do with a rich man stealing a poor man's only sheep. David was outraged by the man's sin; ironically, Nathan told this story to expose the king's sin. David was so disconnected from his sin that although he could recognize sin in others, he could not see it in himself. He had lived in denial too long!

5. Damaging Consequences. The son born to David and Bathsheba died. Denial and its resulting deception are always damaging.

God's Reality Check

Praise our magnificent Father above that He pursues us despite denial and deception. In David's case, Nathan confronted the king with his sin: " 'You are the man!' " (2 Sam. 12:7). What a shock for the king! This type of exposure can be excruciatingly painful. But we see the heart of David when he said, " 'I have sinned against the Lord' " (v. 13). He turned from his denial and back to God.

✻ Read Psalm 51. What evidence did David give that he was no longer in denial? Check the responses that apply.
   ❑ He blamed others for his actions.   ❑ He asked forgiveness.
   ❑ He explained his unusual circumstances.   ❑ He denied involvement.
   ❑ He had a broken and repentant heart.

Denial is woven into the fabric of the human soul because of sin. A personal relationship with Christ offers the opportunity to know truth from God's perspective. Jesus serves as a crystal-clear mirror that offers an accurate reflection of who we really are. All we need to do is ask Him to "search us," as David later did, and He will (Ps. 139:23-24). Knowing Christ and His truth gives us the power to change.

PRACTICE SELF-CONTROL

Paul offered a good starting point for managing our emotions in Galatians 5:22-23 when he concluded his list of the fruit of the Spirit with self-control. Self-control originates with God. God does not ask us to control ourselves by a sheer act of our wills. Instead, He wants us to turn to Him, confessing our inability to control even the smallest aspects of our lives—especially our emotions. Confession—not striving for control—gives the Holy Spirit the opportunity to work in our lives.

God wants us to partner with Him. Although He offers the power of self-control, He requires our cooperation. The spirit in us must be willing. We must want to please Him more than we want to please ourselves. Saying no to temptation is really saying yes to our loving Heavenly Father.

Self-control is a God-given capacity for saying no at the right times. We can identify areas of our lives that reflect self-control. Some of us can say no to sugary desserts because we prefer salty snacks. Others can say no to alcohol or tobacco without a second thought. Still others have no qualms about quitting work on time. Workaholism is not a temptation for them.

"The fruit of the Spirit is love, joy, peace, patience, kindness, goodness, faithfulness, gentleness and self-control."
—Galatians 5:22-23

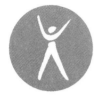

UPREACH

For our purposes, we might re-name self-control *God-control*. Do you ask God for control when you feel your emotions could easily be out of control? For the rest of this week, make a conscious effort to ask God for His control.

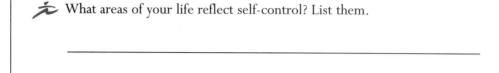 What areas of your life reflect self-control? List them.

_____

_____

Most of us have areas of our lives that could use a dose of self-control. Are you ever tempted to watch television late into the night? Is it a struggle to turn off the computer? Do you crave food or overindulge in spectator sports? You may be asking, "What does this have to do with emotional health?" Emotions must be controlled, just as other areas of life need control. When you learn self-control in one area of life, that discipline is more easily transferred to other areas. So controlling your food intake or television watching really does pay off in terms of controlling your temper or avoiding a pity party.

If you have not seen emotional control modeled in your family of origin, choose friends who seem to maintain good emotional health. Spend time with them. We learn a lot by imitating good behavior.

We have looked at two extremes of emotional imbalance. Emotionally healthy people learn to balance their emotions. They do not deny or deaden their emotions nor do they permit their emotions to rule and dominate their lives. Strike a healthy balance between these two extremes. Instead of denying a feeling of anxiety, for example, allow it to motivate you to reach a difficult goal. Instead of indulging anger, let it work for you positively as you take constructive actions to correct the situation. Most emotions can be successfully balanced.

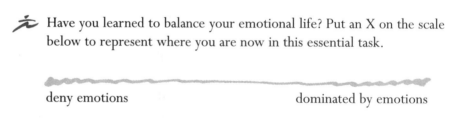 Have you learned to balance your emotional life? Put an X on the scale below to represent where you are now in this essential task.

deny emotions   dominated by emotions

PRACTICE SOLITUDE AND STILLNESS

The busyness of life itself is detrimental to emotional health. I've heard it said this way, "You can't go Mach II speed in a camel body." The statement humorously points out how our bodies are incapable of handling such a fast pace. Like the body, our emotions are hit hard by an intense lifestyle. Too much too fast results in what I call *emotional meltdown*. The meltdown can manifest itself in emotional numbness or over-sensitivity. Either way, the person has exhausted emotional reserves. The person must replenish and fill up!

At different points in church history, the disciplines of solitude and stillness were highly prized and practiced. I understand why they are such oddities today. Who has time for being still when all we know is "Go, Go!" and "Do, Do!"? Who would believe that doing what looks like nothing would produce something positive?

Slow Down and Sit at Jesus' Feet

In Luke 10 one person had an emotional meltdown and another person demonstrated how to replenish her emotional tank. Jesus was visiting the home of Lazarus, Martha, and Mary, His dear friends. He frequently went there to get away from the press of the crowds. As the story progresses, you will see that being close to Jesus does not make a person immune to emotional meltdowns. Martha, busily preparing their meal, got so stressed that she ran out of emotional resources. Here are some characteristics of those who have emptied their emotional tanks.

1. They are distracted with too much activity. What was it that distracted Martha? Serving Jesus! Her problem had to do with the way she was going about her relationship to Christ. Serving Christ will never substitute for intimacy with Christ. As a matter of fact, intimacy with Christ will produce service in the form of an easy yoke and a light burden (see Matt. 11:28-30). Religious activity should never prevent you from being with Jesus.

2. They fuss at Jesus. Martha gave Jesus a piece of her mind. She told Him that He must not "care" about her. Although intimacy with God allows us to be honest with our Savior, emotional meltdowns nearly always distort our view of God. Martha viewed Jesus as non-compassionate, maybe insensitive. When your emotions are fried, your thoughts and perceptions of reality are easily skewed. I believe that is what happened to Martha.

 Read 1 Peter 5:7 in the margin. Underline the words that prove that Martha's charge against Jesus was wrong.

3. They feel alone and deserted. Martha complained that she was doing all the work while her sister was not helping. I noticed this same characteristic in myself during the old days of "frenzied activity." I would be sweating over a task and get the sense that I was the only one in the whole world who was doing a thing. I would say under my breath, "Why am I the only one working?" in a self-righteous way. Like Martha, I could only see what I was doing.

4. They can be demanding. Martha's words to Jesus were: " 'Tell her [Mary] to help me!' " (Luke 10:40). When one is overly busy, the goal becomes to get others to speed up also. The assumption is that busyness and fast-paced living are correct, so everyone else should fall in line. In reality Martha needed to slow her pace.

Jesus loved Martha and responded to her, "Martha, Martha" (Luke 10:41-42). He was not upset at her. He knew she needed help, so He told her several things.

1. Too many things should never crowd out the "main thing." The many things pulling at Martha were not as important as the one thing her sister Mary was doing—sitting at His feet and listening to His words. I don't believe Jesus is against activity or balanced busyness. I think Jesus was saying that being with Him comes before serving Him. Being with Him empowers one for service. How easy it is to put busyness ahead of being with Christ.

OUTREACH
Have you ever thought that time alone might be the best thing you can do to improve your relationships with others? Try it today.

"Cast all your anxiety on him because he cares for you."
—1 Peter 5:7

2. You have a choice about how you run your life. Jesus told Martha that Mary had chosen the best part. The word *chosen* indicates that we choose how we spend our time. Jesus wanted Martha to choose intimacy with Him.

Deciding to slow down is the most drastic change I have ever made. Like Martha, I was a "doer," and a pretty good one if I do say so myself. Yet it got me in trouble in the long haul. An emotional meltdown resulted in a clinical depression. My emotions were in such horrible shape that I had to learn to do life differently. A part of doing life differently was making stillness and solitude with Christ a priority.

At first I could only tolerate short periods of stillness before I would have to go "do" something, but gradually I extended the time. Now I long to be with Him. I hunger for His presence. It is as if I am not the same person I used to be. I don't want to make it sound easy, because it is not. Yet, I have a choice to make. Will I enter the rat race, or will I choose a less-traveled road? I choose the path that leads to rich intimacy with Jesus. Part of that path is making time for our relationship.

 In what ways are you like Martha? In what ways are you like Mary?

I am like Mary when I ... _____

I am like Martha when I ... _____

What would have to happen for you to be more intentional about sitting at Jesus' feet and hearing His words?

_____

_____

Solitude and stillness are crucial to growing into full maturity in faith—and to emotional maturity as well. Emotional wellness requires pulling away occasionally for time spent alone in reflection and meditation. We know that quiet time increases our spiritual sensitivity and reduces physical signs of stress. Perhaps it is a new thought for you that quiet time also helps to promote emotional balance.

 Do you have a place where you can get away for moments of solitude and stillness? If so, write your plan for how you will use this place to refresh yourself emotionally. If not, what can you do to create such a place? List your ideas.

_____

_____

> "Very early in the morning, while it was still dark, Jesus got up, left the house and went off to a solitary place, where he prayed."
> —Mark 1:35

JOURNAL THOUGHTS AND PRAYERS

When you began this class, you were given an *Accountability Journal* to record your food and exercise choices. Do you regularly write something under the heading

"Thoughts for the Day"? If so, you are already journaling! If not, begin with these few lines as a good introduction to the practice of journaling. When you become comfortable with journaling, you will need more room to write. Some people invest in a nice decorative notebook, but a spiral-bound tablet will do fine.

Journaling for over 20 years has made a tremendous difference in my relationship to Christ and in my emotional health. Let me share several benefits of journaling.

1. Writing my thoughts has helped me slow down and really think. I frequently found my mind racing or wandering. Writing allowed my mind to quiet its pace and helped me stay on track.
2. The journal provides a powerful tool for me to "cry out" to God; for me to say, "I can't!"; for me to admit my "desperation." It is healing and cleansing.
3. It makes me accountable to my commitment to periods of solitude and stillness. All I need to do is look at the last dated page to see how long it has been since I last spent time alone away from my regular schedule.
4. It provides me with a detailed look at my emotional, spiritual, mental, and physical journey. As I look through it, I get a sense of who I am and where I have been. I can see patterns of behavior, victories, and progress.

Here are some guidelines for effective journaling.

- Journaling has no power in itself. Writing on a tablet or in a journal is not magic. LeAnne Payne says journaling "is a way of keeping track of what we say to God and what we hear Him say."[1]
- Journaling may be done in many different ways. Feel free to journal in a way that is most helpful for you. At times I write out prayers, and at other times I record the events of the day. Find what best works for you. Experiment.
- Record insights you get from reading the Bible and other helpful resources. The Bible is God's life manual for us. Steadily taking in His word is essential for emotional healing and growth.
- Record in the journal what God tells you. This might be a specific Bible verse or passage, but it could also be thoughts and perceptions. We can ask God to teach us to know His voice. His voice will never violate the written Word of God. There are many other voices out there (such as Satan's and the world's).

Keep your journal indefinitely to have a clear, long-term record of your emotional growth. Look back at previous entries occasionally. You will discover answers to prayers that you may have prayed years before. Reviewing your journal can encourage your faith walk.

 If you are an experienced journaler, be prepared to share with your group benefits you have found from journaling.

LOOK TO GOD

We need God! You must be thinking, *Of course I know I need God! I wouldn't be in this study if God were not important to me.* Allow me to explain. When I think of needing God, I think of other things I believe I need such as friends, food, money, and success. Yet our need for God is different. You see, we must have God!

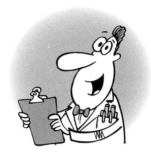

Professor Phitt says:

Analyze your exercise entries in your *Accountability Journal*. Are you getting a variety of exercise: strength training, flexibility, and aerobic exercises? Review pages 14-17 in your *Journal* to develop a F.I.T.T. plan.

INREACH

Think of a specific answer to prayer you have received recently. If you are not presently keeping a journal, record this answer under "Thoughts for the Day" in your *Accountability Journal* entry for today.

A few years ago I did not realize how desperately I needed God. For the most part, I was able to survive with just enough of God to make me feel comfortable and cozy, but not enough to truly transform my life. Then it happened! Life fell in on me, and I could no longer get along with just a little bit of God. I needed Him as never before. That was when I realized I must have Him, and when all I had was God, He was enough. I would like to give you three short phrases that God used to awaken and expand my need for Him: I can't; God can; I want Him to.

I Can't!

Paul said he was not sufficient if left alone. He had learned to say *I can't!* Jesus said, " 'without Me you can do nothing' " (John 15:5, NKJV). God told Paul, " 'My strength is made perfect in weakness.' " Paul concluded, "when I am weak, then I am strong" (2 Cor. 12:9-10, NKJV). We were not created to function on our own. We are invited to lean on Christ for all that we do. Don't expect the world to affirm you when you admit *I can't!* It is cross-cultural—maybe out of this world. I don't believe you can wholeheartedly say *God can!* if you don't first say *I can't!*

God Can!

God is the One who gave a child to barren Sarah; parted the Red Sea and drowned the Egyptians; defeated thousands of Midianites through Gideon and a few men; protected the three Hebrew boys from Nebuchadnezzar's fiery furnace; shut the mouths of lions for Daniel; walked on the water and fed thousands with a little. He is the One who overcame death and the grave. Yes, He can!

I Want Him To!

Saying, *I want You to ...* lets God know that we are ready and willing for Him to do what we can't. In 2 Corinthians 3:6 (NKJV) Paul said God makes us "sufficient." The phrase allows us to turn away from ourselves and to God as the answer to our problem or dilemma. We can trust God to heal our emotions, overcome our self-ishness, or empower us to forgive one who has hurt us deeply.

These three phrases allow us to take incremental steps toward deepening dependency on our Savior, Jesus Christ. The end result will be emotional growth.

 Let's practice these three steps now. In a quiet place, ask God to bring to your mind a relationship, emotion, or another situation that is too diffi-cult for you to handle alone. Take this situation through each of the three steps: I can't; God can; I want Him to! Do not rush. Allow God time to move in your heart and speak to you.

As you close for the week, can you list in the margin the five suggestions for man-aging emotions? If not, turn back to the beginning of the chapter to review.

"Not that we are competent in ourselves to claim anything for ourselves, but our competence comes from God. He has made us competent as ministers of a new covenant."
—2 Corinthians 3:5-6

Managing Emotions

1.

2.

3.

4.

5.

[1]Leanne Payne, *Listening Prayer* (Grand Rapids, Mich.: Baker Books, 1994), 19.

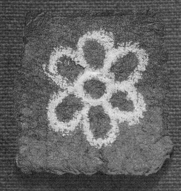

Week Seven

Motivating Yourself

In his book *Emotional Intelligence,* Daniel Goleman encourages us to consider the positive motivation we get from emotions—"the marshaling of feelings of enthusiasm, zeal, and confidence."[1] These feelings lead to achievement of our goals. Too often I have experienced the opposite of what Goleman describes. Rather than being able to use my emotions to motivate myself, I found they were barriers to achieving my goals. Until just a few years ago, I felt that my emotions and I were on opposing teams. I wanted to be excited about each day and all God had for me, but my emotions refused to cooperate with my direction.

Allowing our emotions to motivate us is like the wind that drives the sail to move us in a given direction. You can row your boat without wind, but it is much easier to make progress if you harness the power of the wind. Rowing can be compared to struggling to force our emotions to cooperate. We make progress in reaching our goals, but the struggle is very tiring. The wind is an illustration of our being able to use our emotions to reach our goals—getting our emotions on our team.

 Do you feel your emotions are on your team or on the opposing team? (Check one.)

❑ My team   ❑ The opposing team

Frequently, we allow our emotions to lead us rather than to give direction to our emotional expression. We act based on those feelings before we have applied our minds and our spirits to the issue at hand. Emotions must work in tandem with mind, soul, and body for us to experience emotional wellness. (For additional information on mental, spiritual, and physical wellness, see *With all my Mind: God's Design for Mental Wellness* (0-6300-0584-3); *With all my Soul: God's Design for Spiritual Wellness* (0-6300-0585-1); and *With all my Strength: God's Design for Physical Wellness* (0-6300-0586-X). See page 95 for ordering information.

This week we will look at ways to enlist our minds, souls, and bodies in getting our emotions on our team. Then we will examine the process by which we make appropriate changes.

ENGAGE YOUR MIND

Recall from week 1 that our emotions have a mental component. What we tell ourselves, the facts we feed our brains, and our belief systems affect our emotions. For example, if I tell myself I will never be a worthwhile person until I achieve some great accomplishment, I may find myself in a mid-life crisis at age 50. If I believe that only thin people are attractive, I may go into an emotional dive if I put on a few extra pounds.

We have a great capacity to control our thoughts, just as we have the ability to manage our emotions. A diet of television sitcoms and romance novels does not nourish mental alertness or discernment. Challenge your brain with new information. Feed your mind positive thoughts.

 Read the words of Paul in the margin. Underline words that describe what we are to think about. What thoughts does this Scripture rule out?

_____

"Finally, brothers, whatever is true, whatever is noble, whatever is right, whatever is pure, whatever is lovely, whatever is admirable—if anything is excellent or praiseworthy—think about such things."
—Philippians 4:8

Choose the Good, Realizing Your Emotions Will Follow

Our emotions were not indended to rule. We are to be God-controlled, not emotions-controlled. If I wake up in a bad mood, I don't have permission to take it out on you. I can choose to act toward you with *agape* love despite my bad mood. Far from being insincere or manipulative, acting in love demands a high degree of commitment and perseverance. It requires us to act as we believe we are called to act, rather than being the victim of our moods or feelings. A*gape* love acts lovingly even when human standards might otherwise give us permission to be unloving.

Brad tended to be impatient with his children. When he taught them a skill, he had difficulty waiting for their little fingers to perform simple tasks. Often Brad found himself yelling at them, as though that would make the task go faster. Brad determined to act as if he were patient. Each time he became frustrated by his children's clumsiness, he would ask himself how a patient person would handle the situation. Then he would act accordingly. Over a period of time, Brad became more patient with his children. As an added benefit, he also found himself more patient with his employees.

Perhaps if I am in a bad mood or feeling angry or impatient, I can learn to tell you how I feel and enlist your support and prayers. I do not get to take it out on you!

Act Based on Fact

Often we react emotionally as though we have no facts to guide our decisions. When we internalize God's Word and use it as the foundation for our behavior, we can choose our actions. In her book *Women and Their Emotions*, Miriam Neff says, "Since it is popular to believe there are no absolutes, we ought not to be surprised to find that people act based on feeling; facts have been discredited, and the foundation they once trusted has been made to appear faulty, as the foundation of truth, God's absolute, is hacked and chopped."[2] Emotions were never intended to be the basis for actions. Actions are to be determined by God's absolute truth. Actions begin in our minds. Feelings add vibrancy and color to our lives, but they never should be solely in charge.

 Explain how our emotions are influenced by positive actions.

_____

_____

ENGAGE YOUR SOUL

In week 1 we learned that our emotions have a spiritual component. The psalmist and the prophets often asked God to direct their thoughts and actions. They also prayed for emotional control. "I was overcome by trouble and sorrow. Then I called on the name of the Lord," said the psalmist in Psalm 116:3-4.

In week 6 we determined that emotional control is really God-control. He wants to be Lord of our emotions as well as Lord of our thoughts and actions. Two words that describe the spiritual motivators of our lives are *hope* and *optimism.*

Express Hope

For Christians, hope is much more than wishful thinking. It is more like a guarantee. The assurance of this guarantee is not based on us but on the character of God who cannot lie (Num. 23:19). God will be faithful to the end!

Biblical hope is not wishful thinking but the assurance of what we have not yet seen. The apostle Paul explained to the church at Rome the development of hope: "Hope does not disappoint, because the love of God has been poured out in our hearts by the Holy Spirit who was given to us" (Rom. 5:5, NKJV). He said that tribulation produces perseverance; and perseverance, character; and character, hope. In other words, we can't operate out of hope unless character has been built in us; and character is built on tribulation. The seed of hope is planted in the soil of tribulation.

Tribulation is not the best possible news to those who only want relief from troubles. But if you want God instead of relief, this is great news! Tribulation invites a deep, abiding intimacy with God, resulting in a hope that does not disappoint. Just the thought of that statement overwhelms me.

Cota, my daughter Chelsea's Pembroke Welsh Corgi, provides us with a good example of hope. One day I returned home from town with Cota and Lobo, our Labrador Retriever, in the back of my small pick-up. I went to the back of the truck and opened the tailgate to let the dogs out. Lobo jumped out, but Cota was not there! My heart raced as my son Chase joined me in my search for Cota. We quickly sped off to hunt for our little buddy. As I pulled out of the first side street and onto a major thoroughfare, my son said, "There he is!" What a welcome sight. Cota was in the median running up and down the 50 yards of grass, his small head

UPREACH
While it is true that disappointments come our way, the source of those disappointments is not God. The next time you suffer a disappointment, pause and thank God that He gives us the hope that does not disappoint. In Him, we find encouragement and strength to go on living, caring, and serving.

looking around expectantly. Yes, he was looking for us. He knew we were coming back! Now that is hope!

Endurance and perseverance allow us to continue in the face of tremendous hardship and difficulties. Persons who hope in the Lord know that the Heavenly Father holds the answer. And, He holds onto them!

🏃 Read the following Scriptures and explain the source of hope in each.

Isaiah 41:10 _____

Daniel 3:16-17 _____

Hebrews 12:1-3 _____

In Psalm 43:5, the psalmist said, "Why are you downcast, O my soul? Why so disturbed within me? Put your hope in God, for I will yet praise him, my Savior and my God." His two questions, "Why are you downcast?" and "Why so disturbed within me?" describe his emotions as though they were set in battle array against him. The resounding answer to this problem is to hope in God. In other words, believe that God is good and a better day is coming. Using our emotions to motivate us in positive directions requires that we are anchored deeply in God, the bedrock of hope. Pray the following prayer along with me or write one of your own in the margin.

> *Father, thank You that problems and pains do not have to hamper my relationship with You. In fact, they can motivate me to trust You more. Give me eyes that see problems from Your perspective. You are good and can make all things work together for good for us who love You and who have been called according to Your purpose. Bring this to pass, Father. Amen.*

Learn to Be Optimistic

A popular word for *hope* is *optimism*. Why does one person see a cup half-full and another, observing the same cup, declares it half-empty? A cartoon offers an example of this difference in human personality. A young boy and girl are observing an ambulance going down the street with its lights flashing. In the next frame the little boy sadly says, "Somebody is hurt." In the following frame the girl says, "Somebody is getting help." What a contrast. The little girl viewed her world through the eyes of optimism.

A realistic optimist experiences many positive emotions. They believe everything is going to work out, that good will come from the experience. They are fully aware of set backs and disappointments. However, they have the capacity to see beyond the present problems to a positive solution or a better day. Of all people, Christians should be the most optimistic because of the hope promised in Christ.

"We know that in all things God works for the good of those who love him, who have been called according to his purpose."
—Romans 8:28

Often, pessimists—those who expect the worst-case scenario and are surprised when life flows smoothly—simply operate out of learned behavior. Perhaps a parent or significant other was a pessimist. Children learn to imitate the adults in their lives. Research has shown that a pessimist can become an optimist by training his or her mind to react positively to daily events.

 Explain how an optimist and a pessimist would react to each of the following activities.

A long car trip

An optimist would say_____

A pessimist would say_____

An afternoon rain shower

An optimist would say_____

A pessimist would say_____

A registered letter

An optimist would say_____

A pessimist would say_____

Analyze Your View of God

Beliefs about God play significant roles in individuals' levels of hope and optimism. Let's look at some commonly-held but inaccurate views of God.

1. A Demanding God. Persons who see God as demanding view Him as never being pleased with them or anything they do. No matter what they do or how hard they try to develop a relationship with God, these persons perceive that God's response will always be, "You could have tried a little harder," or "You just never do anything right!" Their view of God is nearly always accompanied by feelings of rejection and discouragement.

2. An Angry God. The small black puppy lay cowering on the ground in front of me. He seemed to be communicating, "Please don't kick me." As I walked on, I noticed he cowered before everyone who approached him. He expected all humans to be angry and to hurt him. This puppy's reaction is not much different from the person who sees God primarily as angry and vengeful. This view of God creates a strong feeling of fear, which may be expressed as worry and anxiety—or in extreme forms, paranoia about God "getting them."

3. A Distant God. "God never seems very real to me," Ben said to his student minister. "I get the sense that He created everything, flung it into space, turned His back, and walked away. I have never really been able to connect

A pessimist can become an optimist by training the mind to react positively to daily events.

61

with God. I suppose it will always be this way." Ben seemed convinced that God is always aloof and detached. Having this view of God can result in feeling abandoned. It is the sense of being truly alone in the world.

4. A Powerless God. These persons see God as unable to change a situation or unable to empower them to cope with it. They think God's power is limited. They see God as wanting to help but being unable to do so. This view of God results in feelings of hopelessness. Continuation of this hopelessness can lead to despair.

Do you identify with one of these views? If so, place a star beside it in the margin. Underline the resulting emotions you feel. If you do not identify with these views of God, describe how your view affects your feelings.

My view: _____

Its Effect: _____

ENGAGE YOUR BODY

Jesus said it well, " 'The spirit is willing, but the body is weak' " (Matt. 26:41). In week 1 we found that the body plays a significant role in emotional expression. If we are too tired, too hungry, or too stressed, our emotions will often be out of control. A physical check-up is a great way to begin a plan for emotional wellness.

Taking care of our bodies through rest and proper nourishment helps us implement our plans. Engaging the mind and soul will be inadequate if we suffer from sleep deprivation and vitamin or mineral deficiency.

You may be saying, *How can I get everything done if I take time for these things?* I wrestle with the same feelings. Our rat-race society convinces us that more is better and the faster the better. More activity is not the answer to emotional wellness, while taking care of my mind, soul, and body is essential to it. We've talked before about how we get our emotions on our team. Total wellness is emotions, minds, spirits, and bodies working together and not in isolation.

Fit 4 is based on Jesus' admonition that we love God with our hearts, souls, minds, and strength. Which of these best complete the statement for you?

My heart, soul, mind and strength …
❑ all work together well.
❑ are making progress in working together.
❑ are unequal. One is winning over the others.
❑ are at war with each other.
❑ Other_____

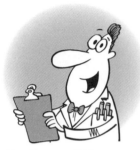

Professor Phitt says:

Muscle is very active tissue that burns calories. Consistent resistance training can increase muscle tissue and/or prevent age-related muscle loss, thereby boosting and retaining your body's ability to burn more calories even at rest. Resistance training exercises include using weights, resistance tubing or bands, and swimming or water exercise.

Choose one of the dark emotions from week 2 (see pages 22-23).
Explain how you can turn this emotion into a motivator in a given situation. Be prepared to share your answer with your group.

Emotion: _____

Situation: _____

How it can motivate: _____

THE CHANGE PROCESS

Often we sincerely desire to use emotional energy to positively motivate us, but our good intentions fail. Our "want to" is too tied up in circumstances and feelings. Miriam Neff raises this issue in her book, *Women and Their Emotions.*

> How do you capture an octopus? Do you grab one leg and tuck it under your arm, hoping the other seven tentacles don't strangle you before you capture another? …We sometimes wrestle with our emotions this way. We decide we must tackle one area, let's say, anger. We work at it for weeks. Maybe we even see some progress. But, meanwhile, we get jealous of someone who never has to wrestle with anger because he is such a docile person. Maybe we decide we'll take on loneliness and depression and deal with them in one grand program of activity. … But in the bustle of activity we find insecurity stalking us, messing up or tangling our well-laid plans. It's hard to battle inadequacies, loneliness, and depression if insecurity has our hands tied behind our backs.[3]

If you have participated in the *Fit 4 Nutrition* course, you are familiar with the change process, taken from my book with James Porowski, *Strength for the Journey* (LifeWay Press: 0-7673-9105-5). Let me review it for you.

1. Develop awareness. Change is necessary when you realize that some aspect of your lifestyle is not working for you or could work better. God makes us aware of these needed changes through other people, circumstances, or His Word. Denial is the opposite of awareness. Staying in denial keeps us from realizing the benefits that occur through positive changes. Fortunately, when God asks you to change, He gives you the power, but you must agree to partner with Him. (*Fit 4* Nutrition *Member Workbook,* p. 24)

2. Gain knowledge. Occasionally, we know the steps to take to implement our awareness of a needed change. Sometimes we need more information. For example, we may know that sugar and caffeine are keeping us from getting sleep, but we may need information on how to read food labels to detect these substances. We may know a relationship needs restoring through forgiveness, but we may not know the way to go about re-establishing contact. Talking with a Christian counselor can provide an understanding of how to accomplish the goal. (*Fit 4* Nutrition *Member Workbook,* p. 25)

INREACH

Let's practice this process. Select an emotion that you would like to cultivate to motivate positive actions such as optimism, perseverance, or patience. Apply the four steps of the change process during the next 30 days. Cultivate the habits that encourage the expression of this emotion. In your *Accountability Journal* or another notebook, chart your progress. Be willing to share your experience with a trusted friend, your facilitator, or your group.

OUTREACH

Share the change process with a friend, family member, or coworker who you know is seeking to modify a behavior. You will encourage him or her in the wellness journey.

3. Take action. You can be aware that change is necessary and gain valuable information, but if you never act on this knowledge, you will not change. Habits are formed by repeating an action. Studies show that 21 to 30 days of repetition make an action a habit, and six months' repetition incorporates it into your lifestyle. (***Fit 4*** *Nutrition Member Workbook,* p. 26)

4. Experience change. New habits and lifestyle choices must be maintained in order to produce lasting good. ***Fit 4*** is a plan for a lifetime, not a time-out from your regular routine. Change does not equal perfection, but it does mean that over time you act on more of the new behaviors than the old behaviors. (***Fit 4*** *Nutrition Member Workbook,* p. 27)

Let's consider the story of Peter's vision in Acts 10 as a change model. God gave Peter a vision instructing him three times to eat unclean food (awareness). Peter was so repulsed that he initially rejected the whole idea. By asking Peter to do what God's law forbade, God used this vision to convince Peter that the Gentiles were to be saved along with the Jews (knowledge). Peter then went to the home of a Gentile, Cornelius, and baptized him (action). Then Peter explained his actions to his Jewish friends (change). It took much convincing to persuade staunch Jews that Jesus' free gift of salvation extended beyond God's chosen nation. God desires to include all of us in His plan (Rom. 1:16).

Peter's change process was not perfect (see Gal. 2:11-14). Taking a backward step should not discourage us from continuing the change process. There will be more forward than backward steps if we persist in acting on the new behaviors.

Turn to page 24 and review the goals which you set for this study. Below list actions you have taken that indicate that your awareness and knowledge are leading you to change.

Actions: _____

_____

_____

---

[1]Daniel Goleman, *Emotional Intelligence* (New York: Bantam, 1995), 79.
[2]Miriam Neff, *Women and Their Emotions* (Chicago: Moody Press, 1983), 18.
[3]Ibid., 15.

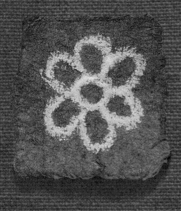

Developing Relationships

VERSE TO KNOW

"Dear friends, let us love
one another, for love
comes from God."
—1 John 4:7

"How does Tony make friends so easily?" Bill asked John.

"Tony makes people feel accepted and comfortable in his presence," John replied. "They really enjoy being with him."

Bill walked away from the conversation, wishing he could be as good at relationships as his friend Tony. "It must be a special gift," he concluded.

Relationship skills are not just mystery—some have it and some don't. All of us can improve our ability to interact with others. As a young boy growing up in the piney woods of East Texas, I frequently heard my mom say to us children, "You have got to learn to get along!" She wanted us to fuss with each other less and play more cooperatively. Mom's statement, "You have got to learn to get along!" is a simple way of saying we needed to mature in the way we related to each other.

Recall that emotions are the voice of relationships. In order for us to be emotionally well, we must avoid habits that stifle relationships and embrace those that enhance relationships.

HABITS THAT STIFLE RELATIONSHIPS

Six habits will stifle, if not destroy, relationship development.

Talking Too Little

As you can well imagine, the one who talks too little has tremendous difficulty maintaining one-on-one conversation. Often this type person will congregate in groups of people so as to camouflage his or her inability to communicate. Talking too little may be a way of hiding out from others or a form of passive aggression: "You want me to talk? Well, forget it!" If you need to learn to carry your end of the conversation, remember that practice makes perfect. Ask questions of the other person as a way to begin talking more.

"Do not let any unwholesome talk come out of your mouths, but only what is helpful for building others up according to their needs, that it may benefit those who listen."
—Ephesians 4:29

INREACH
Take this test of bravery:
Ask a close friend to evaluate your non-verbal communication (what you do with your eyes, face, hands, and so forth).
Express thanks for the input and begin the process of change, if needed (see pp. 63-64).

Talking Too Much

When you are with a person who talks too much, you have to wrestle the conversation away from the other person before you can say anything. This struggle feels somewhat like fighting with a six-year-old for the controls of a video game. After trying for a while to converse with one who monopolizes, you will come to feel you are unnecessary. Often you will listen politely for a few moments longer, and when he or she slows down to gulp in air, you quickly excuse yourself. At this point the person who talks too much moves on to find another victim. This cycle is endless. If you suffer from hyperactivity of the mouth, do as I suggested to those who talk too little—learn to ask your listener questions.

Talking Only About Yourself

"Let me tell you about my new house." "You won't believe what my grandchild did!" "I have one of those, and it is faster." These phrases are trademarks of those who make themselves the center of the conversation. How much or how little they talk is not the problem. The problem is the subject of their talk: me and mine. This one-way relationship will last as long as you can tolerate the other's self-centeredness. Again, asking questions of others helps break this cycle.

Not Listening

This individual is like a radio tower that sends out information but is not concerned with receiving information. For relationships to develop, both parties must transmit and receive data. Receiving data tells the sender if the transmitted message was understood.

Good listening is difficult because it forces you to get out of your frame of reference. Empathy enables you to hear clearly and accurately the words of another. The inability to listen results in shallow, unfulfilling relationships. If you have a tendency to think about something else rather than listen, review the listening skills on page 47.

Distracting Non-Verbal Communication

The words you speak make up a very small percentage of communication. The majority of communication is done at a non-verbal level: voice tone, facial expression, and body posture. When you are relating to another, you consciously hear their words and unconsciously notice their non-verbals.

Most people are not aware of the impact of non-verbals on their relationships. For instance, a smile can mean approval, but no facial expression can mean disinterest. Arms crossed can be a way of distancing oneself. Non-verbal communication that seems to distract from the relationship can be confusing, even if the person says the right words. The only sure way to know what non-verbals mean is to ask.

Becoming aware of these five barriers to effective relationship development will provide a solid foundation for emotional growth.

Evaluate your relationship skills. Beside each of the five habits below indicate where you think you rate by choosing the number that most accurately represents you. Choosing 1 means this characteristic is infrequent in your life and 5 means this characteristic is very common.

talking too little	1	2	3	4	5
talking too much	1	2	3	4	5
talking only about yourself	1	2	3	4	5
not listening	1	2	3	4	5
distracting non-verbal communication	1	2	3	4	5

Using Coping Styles for Protection or Control

Although we seek to cope with life situations in many ways, coping styles can be compressed into three foundational approaches. We learn each of the three during childhood as a way of handling relationship rejection and painful emotions. Usually, one becomes more primary and another a secondary way of dealing with problem people in our lives. These styles can provide information for you to better understand why you may react as you do.

1. Embracers. Embracers have decided that the best way to navigate turbulent relational waters is by loving and caring for others no matter what. If they love others enough, surely they will get rejected less. They do all in their power to keep from offending others, even denying their own needs. Inferiority is a constant companion, as well as an unhealthy dependency. Embracers hate conflict, so they have been known to ask forgiveness for things they did not do just to keep from fighting. A contemporary term for this style is *codependent*. We'll learn more about codependency in week 9.

2. Attackers. These individuals are the opposites of embracers. They are certain that others intend to thwart their plans or hurt them personally. Here are some descriptors of this style: aggressive, shrewd, dominating, insensitive to the feelings of others, controlling, and manipulative. They shun affection and weakness, are afraid to admit error or imperfection, and pursue prestige. They prefer to be the leader and have everyone else follow. If you were to call attention to any personal weakness, an attacker might easily "blow up" at you. Often attackers are very successful and rise to the top of organizations quickly, leaving a trail of wounded individuals in their paths.

3. Avoiders. The life strategy of an avoider is not to get close to anyone as a way of preventing relational hurt. They have learned that if you get too close to people, rejection may result. Their answer to this dilemma is to distance themselves from others—relational hermits, if you will. Just the thought of someone getting close to them causes anxiety. They are aloof and detached. They have a tendency to deny emotions. If you were to observe avoiders, you would see few indicators of their emotional life.

"Do not make friends with
a hot-tempered man,
do not associate with one
easily angered,
or you may learn his ways
and get yourself ensnared."
—Proverbs 22:24-25

Very few people fit exactly into any one of these categories because they are exaggerations of common tendencies. Most people have adapted and combined traits to form their own unique style. However, each of us has a dominant style by which we function most of the time. We also have a secondary style. This fact does not mean that an embracer is unable to attack or that an avoider never embraces. I am an embracer until you push me too far; then I change into an attacker.

Each of these styles can hinder your relationship with others because they do not encourage open, authentic communication. Each style puts self at the center. These coping styles hinder your relationship with Christ because they are forms of self-protection and control rather than an encouragement for you to look to Christ for protection and control. Ask God to help you understand your style and enable you to trust Him more.

 Circle one answer to each of the following questions:

1. When you feel threatened or insecure, which is your primary relational style?

      embracer   attacker   avoider

2. Which is your secondary style?

      embracer   attacker   avoider

3. How does your style impact your relationships?

      detracts   neutral   enhances

Risking emotional exposure rather than circling the wagons and defending yourself is a learned skill. Like your first venture into the deep end of a swimming pool, it gets easier the more you try it. Sure, you can stay in the shallow end forever, but the big kids go deeper.

HABITS THAT ENHANCE RELATIONSHIPS

The way we communicate is one indicator of emotional maturity. If you want to know how mature I am, then pay attention to how I interact with others, not what I say about my maturity level. Dr. Larry Crabb says, "The clearest evidence that people are living as intended by God is that we relate in ways that promote harmony between ourselves and others who relate similarly. A mature pattern of relating involves whatever actions represent the abandonment of self-protection."[1]

Mature communicators would not have as their primary goal guarding self from hurt. Their authentic, open, and honest communication style would be more free of self-protective mechanisms. More likely they would be purposeful about sharing who they really are and how they really feel, stark contrasts to those who are plastic and pretentious.

Use All the Levels of Communication

God intended us to have relationships that are emotionally satisfying. That is why He gave Himself to us and now lives in us. Communication occurs at five levels, each appropriate in given situations. The problem occurs if we do not use all five levels in normal interactions. As you read the five levels, think about the degree to which you use each one in a typical week.

1. *Cliché* communication is restricted to greetings and comments that express no opinion, feelings, or real information. It is strictly a surface or robotic type of communication, often called hallway talk. ("Hi, how are you?" "Fine, thank you.") If it is a primary communication tool, it allows one to remain safely isolated and alone.

2. *Fact* communication consists of objective and non-personal facts, information, or data analysis. There is no intimate or personal sharing at this level. Emotions expressed tend to be superficial. ("Last night the weatherman said we'd have more rain today. I hope not.") Couples may use this level to arrange schedules and relay family news, but it does not build intimacy if used in isolation of the deeper levels.

3. *Opinion* communication focuses on thoughts. A person shares ideas and opinions that will reveal what he or she really thinks. ("I'm really getting concerned about the garbage on television and what it's doing to young people's minds.") Although thoughts are essential clues into the lives of others, unless you know how they feel, you still have an incomplete picture.

4. *Emotional* communication is the sharing of hopes, fears, likes, dislikes, aspirations, disappointments, joys, sorrows, dreams, failures, desires, stresses, sources of fulfillment, discouragements, and burdens. ("I got passed over again for promotion. I have to admit, getting that higher position meant a lot to me. I'm discouraged with this job.") At this level one shares feelings openly. This level leads to deeper, more meaningful relationships.

5. *Soul-mate* communication is maximum self-disclosure. At this level the person opens up his life like a well-used suitcase and allows the other person to view him as he REALLY is. This is the most vulnerable level of communication, practiced by very few of us. ("I desperately want a child. Wouldn't I make a good parent? I can't seem to be reconciled to life without children of my own.")

Soul-mate communication can only be enjoyed with a few close friends or loved ones. We cannot be intimate with hundreds of people. As a matter of fact, that would constitute inappropriate sharing. Personally, I have five soul mates.

Circle the frequency with which you use the five levels of communication in a typical week. (1 = never; 2 = some; 3 = often)

1. cliché	1	2	3
2. fact	1	2	3
3. opinion	1	2	3
4. emotional	1	2	3
5. soul mate	1	2	3

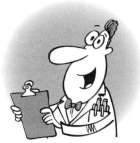

Professor Phitt says:

We often use hallway talk around the water fountain at church or workplace. The next time you get a drink of water, think about asking a question that would take the conversation to a deeper level. By the way, did you know that you need to drink a minimum of 64 ounces of water daily? Check out the *Fit 4* Guidelines for Healthy Eating on page 20 in your *Accountability Journal.*

UPREACH

Loving relationships
are described in
1 Corinthians 13:4-7.
Read these verses. Ask God
to help you demonstrate
your love through
these loving behaviors.

Develop Soul-Mate Relationships

Emotional wellness is impossible to achieve and maintain apart from deep, rich relationships with others. I know how difficult it can be to trust anyone with the delicate pieces of our emotional lives. Many of us have learned that it is safer and easier to keep our emotions to ourselves. Yet God created us with the wonderful capacity to know another in depth. Genesis 2:18 reveals our relational capacity. God said, " 'It is not good for the man to be alone.' " We were designed for intimacy with God and others.

Our *Fit 4* theme verses from Mark 12:30-31 affirm the centrality of relationships in the believer's life. Jesus said the law could be summed up in loving God, your neighbor, and yourself. In John 13:34-35 (NKJV), Jesus said, " 'A new commandment I give to you, that you love one another; as I have loved you, that you also love one another. By this all will know that you are My disciples, if you have love for one another.' " The apostle Paul confirmed this principle in his letter to the Galatians, "For all the law is fulfilled in one word, even in this: 'You shall love your neighbor as yourself' " (5:14, NKJV). Love is at the center of the heart of God. Love is also impossible to maintain without meaningful communication. That is why we are to pray daily in order to maintain an intimate relationship with God.

Emotional growth most readily occurs in the soil of soul-mate relationships. What does a soul-mate relationship look like? If you were to listen in on the dialogue, you would get the sense that talking has become a natural process. The shared unity between the participants makes talking seem easy. You may get the impression that they have known each other for a long time, but it may have only been weeks or months. It may be helpful to look back at pages 65-68 to review some communication barriers that prevent or retard this level of communication. Here are some characteristics of soul-mate relationships.

1. Vulnerable. Most of us have learned that it is not always safe out there in the relational jungle we call life. We have developed ways to protect ourselves from the hurts that others may cause us. I used to feel like one of King Arthur's knights covered from head to toe with thick armor plating. I had the belief that if I wore enough protection I would never be hurt or disappointed again. Not so! Even a turtle must come out of its shell occasionally. We need to take some of that armor off to build the type of relationships that produce emotional health. We relate best to others when they know who we really are and vice-versa. I am not suggesting that you remove all your armor at once and in all situations, but you can remove one piece at a time as certain relationships develop. You will find your Heavenly Father can protect you better than any armor.

2. Purposeful. Relationships that produce emotional health must be built intentionally. They won't happen on their own. You will have to be proactive rather than reactive or passive. If you do not have a soul-mate relationship with anyone, ask God to provide it. This request is a proactive and intentional step toward health. Another thing you can do is go where people are. It is hard to develop depth relationships if you are not around people. Make yourself available to God and others and see what happens.

3. Self-disclosure. I know of no better way to develop a relationship to a soul-mate level than by the use of self-disclosure. It will take time to get comfortable and secure enough to open up in a way that allows the person to see who you really are. Allow God to work at His pace; there is no need to get in a big hurry. When the time comes to share in depth about your life, it will take a little courage. Go ahead, for this is the path to maturity. I remember being a bit anxious and fearful the first few times I shared my heart with another. I hoped that they would accept it and not think badly of me. The more I practiced self-disclosure, the easier it was. The more my relationship with Christ grew, the safer it was to let others see the real me. I was assured of His acceptance no matter how my friend reacted to my self-disclosure. For many of us, self-disclosure will be a big step.

4. Challenge. When you begin to build a close relationship with someone, you can expect to face problems. It seems to be the nature of relationships. You need only thumb through the pages of the Bible to see just how difficult relationships can be. You are in good company! You are on a most wonderful adventure as you grow with others in Christ. Nothing this fulfilling would ever be accomplished without some trials and disappointments. Persevere my brothers and sisters! Our Savior has run the race before us so we need not be dismayed. Endure in your pursuit of soul-mate intimacy, and I promise you will not be disappointed.

Soul-mate relationships give us a ready resource in times of trouble. Often we need help along the way; we need someone to help carry our burdens (Gal. 6:2). The picture painted in this verse is of one who is overburdened with life's problems, unable to free himself alone. That is when God provides the soul-mate. Oh, what a blessing to have one walk alongside us as we journey toward wellness.

OUTREACH

Are you a person someone else could trust with privileged information? To have a friend, be a friend. Take seriously Solomon's warnings against gossip in Proverbs 16:28 and 20:19.

"Carry each other's burdens." —Galatians 6:2

What steps do you need to take this week to begin growing in this area of soul-mate development? Check the actions below that you will take.
- ❑ Pray for a soul mate.
- ❑ Practice levels 3 and 4 (p. 69) on a more consistent basis.
- ❑ Work on relationship skills such as listening and asking questions.
- ❑ Be available to people by going where they are gathered.
- ❑ Practice self-disclosure with a safe person.
- ❑ Be a safe person to someone else.
- ❑ Other

A Biblical Picture of Soul-Mate Relationships

Alan Tomlinson, a colleague of mine, introduced me to a wonderful picture of soul-mate relationships from the Bible. The aged apostle Paul was at the end of his life, imprisoned, and forsaken by some of his friends. What an emotional challenge! Read these words in 2 Timothy 1:16-17 (NKJV), "The Lord grant mercy to the household of Onesiphorus, for he often refreshed me, and was not ashamed of my chain; but when he arrived in Rome, he sought me out very zealously and found me."

The word *refreshed* can mean "resuscitated" or "make alive again." This word can be illustrated by imagining someone who has been in a dry, hot desert for three days with no water. Suddenly, he comes over a sand dune and sees an oasis with palm trees and a spring-fed pool of cool revitalizing water. He runs to the water and dives headlong into it, gulping the water until his stomach can take no more. Then he falls down on the sandy shore of the pool and relaxes. This scene pictures what Onesiphorus's visit meant to Paul. He was revived and invigorated by the presence of this one who loved him.

Many around Paul had deserted him. He mentions two, Phygellus and Hermogenes, who had abandoned him (2 Tim. 1:15). "Demas has forsaken me, having loved this present world" (2 Tim. 4:10, NKJV). Do you get the picture? Paul had many so-called friends and partners turn away from him, and this turning away occurred at a time when Paul needed them the most! Into this scene of darkness and despair walks Onesiphorus—a ray of sunshine on a dark and dismal day.

Onesiphorus traveled 1,200 miles to reach Paul. What a great friend and soul mate! Once he got to Rome he faced more problems in locating his friend. Rome had no street signs to guide him easily to Paul. This meant he possibly had to search for a lengthy time before he ever reached his friend. Onesiphorus's tenacity and perseverance were amazing considering the stigma that imprisonment carried in those days. Unlike the deserters, Onesiphorus cared more about Paul than the opinion of others. What a blessed man!

Paul and Onesiphorus illustrate soul-mate relationships. The two men were so close in Christ that the very presence of one touched the heart and soul of the other. No doubt they had previously had many moments of honest self-disclosure. The Scripture assumes a deep relationship. This passage offers us a window through which to view soul mates in action. What an awesome sight!

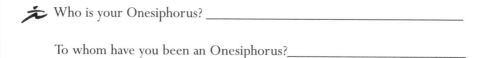 Who is your Onesiphorus? _____

To whom have you been an Onesiphorus?_____

As we close this week's study, pray this prayer with me or write one of your own.

> *Father, You know how scared I am of opening up to other people. I have been hurt by some I thought I could trust. It seems much easier to hide out. But You have made me for relationship. I know that part of my character growth depends on my willingness to go deeper with my communication. Help me to trust You and to find my acceptance in You. I love You with all my heart, soul, mind, and strength. Amen.*

---

[1]Larry Crabb, *Understanding People* (Grand Rapids: Zondervan, 1987), 196.

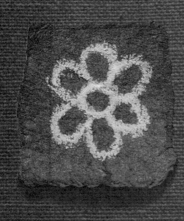

Week Nine

Challenges to Emotional Wellness

During the past eight weeks, we examined emotional wellness: what it looks like in terms of five components and how it relates to God, self, and others (p.41). This week we will look at special challenges to emotional wellness: dark emotions; addictive behaviors such as food addictions and codependency; and perfectionism.

Two strategies will be identified that enable individuals to seek growth and healing from the best source possible: our loving Heavenly Father.

DEALING WITH DARK EMOTIONS

These emotions are labeled *dark* because most people consider them uncomfortable and undesirable. If asked whether they would like a serving of dark emotions, most would answer, *No thanks!* However, dark emotions are normal parts of our everyday experiences. We need to learn to own rather than to deny or disregard them. God allowed His dark emotions (anger and sadness) to be reflected in the Bible. Remember: emotions are! Dark emotions add to the rich emotional expression designed by a loving Creator. However, no emotion should dominate or control us. When dark emotions continually envelope us, we should consider ourselves sidetracked on the journey to emotional wellness.

Discouragement and Depression

Dale was very concerned about his wife, who stayed in bed most of the day. Her appetite was gone; she expressed self-hate and shame. Until recently, she had lots of friends; now she was pulling away from everyone, even Dale. At times Dale was not sure his wife wanted to continue living. He felt helpless and confused.

Dale's wife has symptoms of depression: sleep and eating problems, difficulty concentrating, a vague sense of hopelessness, and despair. Although often used interchangeably, depression is not the same emotion as discouragement. Discouragement lasts a shorter time and is less intense. Some describe it as "feeling blue" or "just a little down." It can end in an hour or a day, whereas depression's symptoms are constant for at least two weeks. Discouraging situations are part of life. In Jesus's words, " 'In the world you will have tribulation' " (John 16:33, NKJV).

"O Lord, God of my salvation,
I have cried out day and night
    before You.
Let my prayer come before You;
Incline Your ear to my cry.
For my soul is full of troubles,
And my life draws near to
    the grave.
I am counted with those who
    go down to the pit;
I am like a man who has no
    strength."
    —Psalm 88:1-4 (NKJV)

"I am so troubled that I cannot
    speak.
Will the Lord cast off forever?
And will He be favorable no
    more?
Has His mercy ceased forever?
Has His promise failed
    forevermore?
Has God forgotten to be
    gracious? …
And I said, 'This is my anguish.' "
    —Psalm 77:4,7-10 (NKJV)

INREACH
The next time you feel guilt
and shame, ask, Is this feeling
originating with God at work
in me through the Holy Spirit,
or have I taken a burden
upon myself that I was
never meant to carry?

 Dark emotions are woven into the fabric of the Psalms. In the margin, underline words of despair and discouragement.

The psalmist's words reveal a person wrestling through discouragement. This dark emotion was experienced by many of God's strongest leaders. If you or someone you know struggles with depression, first get a complete physical check-up. Professional counseling and/or a support group help develop coping skills. For additional information, read *Strength for the Journey* (LifeWay Press, ISBN 0-7673-9105-5).

Fear and Anxiety
When we feel threatened, fear and anxiety strike. Balanced caution is always good. However, anxiety and fear are rarely balanced and less rarely good. Some label our age as the "generation of anxiety." The news media saturates us with the world's woes, resulting in our being aware of problems that we have no means to fix. This sense of helplessness heightens anxiety.

A person "paralyzed by fear" may feel frozen in place, unable to get it off his mind. Fear may keep him from resting and performing daily activities. Such fear takes the focus off God and puts it on self. It affects intimacy with God. Anxiety and fear are normal reactions to an overwhelming causal agent. However, they should not be so common or acute that they disrupt your daily living.

In the Sermon on the Mount, Jesus assured us that worry produces no good return on our investment. It is a direct denial of belief in a loving Heavenly Father who we can trust to provide our needs. (See Matthew 6:25-34.)

Shame and False Guilt
Unrealistic shame and false guilt drive people to drugs, illicit sexual activity, even suicide. Like lepers in Jesus' day, persons feeling shame and false guilt may believe that everyone knows they are "unclean." They may think they have to apologize for existing. They live with tremendous self-hate, feeling worthless. They believe they are beyond forgiveness. Shame and false guilt are ruthless; they take no prisoners.

 What do you think is the difference between guilt and false guilt?

_____

_____

Guilt results from real sin and can be forgiven by God and others that the sin affected. False guilt, though, is assumed out of a need for self-punishment or unrealistic standards. It cannot be forgiven and forgotten because it is false. If a person cannot "forgive" herself because she was not in the room when her mother died, she suffers from false guilt. She has violated no moral law against God.

Anger

I have been in the position of both giving and receiving anger that shows up unannounced and uninvited. At times it seems to have a mind of its own. Once present, it creates havoc, leaving wounded and hurting people in its path. Dallas Willard says that behind anger is a wounded ego and a strong sense of self-righteousness. These two driving forces combine to harm the one who caused the offense. Anger says, "I will get you back! You will pay! I can't wait to see you hurt!"[1] Those who do not release anger turn it in on themselves. Anger turned inward combined with shame can lead to deep discouragement and despairing depression.

Look again at the distinctions between the anger both God and Jesus displayed and the anger we typically show (see pp. 17-18). Self-serving, self-righteous, or vindictive anger becomes a character issue that can only be resolved by allowing the Holy Spirit to give us self-control (see Gal. 5:23). If venting anger in an appropriate manner is an issue for you, consider Christian counseling or an accountability partner to hold you accountable for your words and actions.

Grief

People who experience loss rarely find simple, quick comfort or relief. Grieving people go through cycles of emotions including shock, denial, anger, confusion, and depression—resulting in a sense of emotional imbalance and turbulence.

Shortly after my father died, my daughter Chelsea and I were Christmas shopping. I had the flash thought, *What will I get Dad for Christmas?* The thought lingered for just a moment before reality crashed: *He's gone! He's gone! There will be no more Christmases with him!* The sense of loss and grief gripped me. The finality of death touched every part of my being. Dad was gone, and I could not bring him back. Maybe you or someone close to you has had a similar experience. Grief and loss are common experiences for us, but they are never welcome guests.

 In the margin, read what Jesus said to comfort Martha at her brother Lazarus' grave. What did Paul mean in 1 Thessalonians 4:13 when he told believers not to grieve as those who "have no hope"?

_____

A normal cycle of grief can last two years or longer, but prolonged grief that does not get closer to resolution over a period of time should be another red flag. Christian counseling or a support group can offer invaluable help. For more information, see *Recovering from the Losses of Life* (LifeWay Press, ISBN 0-8054-9874-5).

Doubt and Confusion

If you have ever experienced doubt and confusion, you know they are burdensome and troubling. We know that Thomas, the doubter, was one of Jesus' disciples, but another doubter may surprise you. Matthew 11:2-3 (NKJV) says, "When John (the Baptist) had heard in prison about the works of Christ, he sent two of his disciples and said to Him (Jesus), 'Are You the Coming One, or do we look for another?' "

> "Jesus said to her, 'I am the resurrection and the life. He who believes in me will live, even though he dies; and whoever lives and believes in me will never die.' "
> —John 11:25-26

Now, wait! Didn't John prepare the way for Jesus? Didn't he preach, "Repent, for the kingdom of heaven is at hand!"? (Matt. 3:2, NKJV). Didn't he say, "Behold! The Lamb of God who takes away the sin of the world!"? (John 1:29, NKJV). How could one who was so sure of Jesus have such doubts? I don't have an answer. I only know that no follower of our Lord is immune from the icy grip of doubt.

Doubt can be cleansing and healing when we honestly seek truth—especially in God's Word and with God's people. Doubt and confusion can be debilitating when we suffer in isolation without allowing God to be part of our process. God welcomes honest inquiry (see the Book of Job), but He is not the author of confusion. Read again the Verse to Know (p. 73) and commit it to memory.

ADDICTIVE BEHAVIORS

Addictions are common in our culture. How does a person know if he or she is struggling with an addiction? Here are some symptoms.

- The addiction gives life meaning and purpose. Apart from it, life holds little value.
- Life revolves around the addiction. Relationships are often neglected.
- Emotional pain and intense discomfort occur when away from the addictive substance or relationship (if the addiction is to a person).
- The addiction becomes obsessive; the addict cannot stop thinking about it.
- The addiction numbs pain and helps avoid painful memories or experiences.
- The addiction is used to punish the addict. Low self-esteem or self-hate often leads to self-destructive behavior.

 Look over the previous list. Place a check beside any that may apply to you.

We are destined to be dependent on something or someone for life. Rather than being totally dependent on God, addicts become addicted to something or someone else. The prophet Jeremiah said: "My people have committed two evils: They have forsaken Me, the fountain of living waters, And hewn themselves cisterns—broken cisterns that can hold no water" (2:13, NKJV). Only God can satisfy the insatiable hunger of the human heart. No hand-dug cisterns will do!

Our addictions are not benevolent like our Heavenly Father. Rather than care for us as He does, the addictions destroy us and leave us in ruins. It is time to turn our neediness and dependency over to Christ, the only One who can fulfill and satisfy our souls. Pray the prayer in the margin along with me, or write one of your own.

Food Addictions

Each time Rosie gets upset, she turns to food. Sweets have a soothing effect on her feelings, but the downside is weight gain and health concerns. When she takes time to think about her behavior, Rosie becomes frightened. She wonders whether she is addicted to food. Rosie is not alone. Most food addictions have an emotional component. Food addicts generally learn to deal with emotions by denying, swallowing, or ignoring them as a way to survive. The eating addiction becomes a way to avoid hurtful and painful feelings.

"Godliness with contentment is great gain."
—1 Timothy 6:6

Father, I turn away from all those things that seemed to give me security, meaning, and purpose. I turn to You, the giver of all life. Fill me up with Yourself. Satisfy my hunger and thirst for people and things. Like the woman at the well in John 4, I want the water that will be so satisfying that I will never thirst again. Teach me to recognize when I turn to other sources for satisfaction. I turn from my broken cisterns and turn to You, my Fountain of Living Water. Only You will satisfy. Amen.

The primary food addictions are anorexia, bulimia, and compulsive overeating. The main driver of eating disorders is powerlessness. Food addicts seek control through eating or not eating; body image becomes life's controlling factor. The results are devastating: the more the addict tries to control these areas, the more life gets out of control, eventually becoming unmanageable.

 Following are questions that can help identify persons with food addictions. Put a check beside those you would answer *yes*. One form of denial is to rush through the list because the self-examination is too painful. Ask God to allow you to see yourself clearly and honestly. Pray that you would know His love and acceptance no matter what.

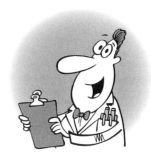

Professor Phitt says:
Eat when you are hungry and stop when you feel full. Eat on a regular schedule. Avoid eating late at night.

Anorexia Nervosa

- (Women) Do you have irregular periods, or have you experienced loss of menstruation for at least three cycles when you otherwise expected it?
- Do you diet to be more slim rather than because you are overweight?
- Do you claim to "feel" fat when others tell you that you are not overweight?
- When others say you are not overweight, do you feel annoyed or irritated, that they are trying to control your body, are jealous, or cannot understand your needs and body?
- Does thinking about food, calories, weight, nutrition, and cooking distract you from other tasks?
- Does physical exercise occupy a disproportionate amount of your time?
- Do you weigh yourself one or more times a day?
- Do you fast, induce vomiting, or use laxatives or diuretics to lose weight?
- Do you hide and hoard food or act out some other type of food-related behavior you think is sensible, but which you prefer others not know?
- Do you feel nauseated or bloated when you eat as much as or less than others your age and size at a normal mealtime (without prior snacking)?
- Do you occasionally binge on food, then feel ashamed and starve yourself?

Bulimia Nervosa

- Are you afraid of being fat, believing that body fat is a sin?
- Do you repeatedly diet, but sabotage your plans by binging and feeling guilt?
- Do you overestimate need for food, especially "oversnacking" under stress?
- Do you hide and hoard private stashes of food for later binging?
- Do you binge on high-calorie, sugary foods or foods such as salads?
- Do you hide your eating (especially binges), fearing scrutiny?
- Do you often feel ashamed and/or depressed when you eat?
- Do you take time from tasks or activities to think about your next binge?
- Do thoughts about food occupy much of your time?
- Does an interruption of this thinking leave you feeling irritable and angry?
- Do you hide these feelings from others?
- Do you use laxatives, diuretics (not prescribed) or exercise to eliminate food you eat or to discharge feelings of anger or anxiety accompanying the binge?
- Do you binge/purge more than three times a week?
- Have you been confronted about and denied your behavior? Did you distance yourself from that person to avoid future confrontations?

Compulsive Overeating

- Are you overweight despite a doctor's and others' prompting to lose weight?
- Have you repeatedly tried to diet, only to fail or sabotage weight loss?
- Do you binge or snack constantly, even while engaging in other activities?
- Do you keep private stashes of snacks, hoping others will not discover them?
- Do you frequently joke in a self-demeaning fashion about your food consumption or body weight?
- Do you go to the trouble of eating alone in secrecy?
- Is food your "friend"?
- Do you have urges to eat when you feel sad, angry, afraid, anxious, or ashamed, or when you experience other unwelcome emotions?
- When you eat, do you think, *I deserve this!?*
- Does shame about your body weight result in additional binges or grazing?
- Do you expend mental energy thinking about food and eating, especially during times when your mind should be focused on other tasks?
- Do you feel angry when interrupted from eating, especially when you're alone?
- As a child, did "Have a cookie" mean "Shut up"? Do you sense that now as well?

OUTREACH

The difference between a caregiver (one who gives appropriate care) and a caretaker (one who takes care of someone else) can be profound. A caretaker may perform functions that keep another person dependent. Underline which word best describes your relationships. For more information on codependency, read *Untangling Relationships: A Christian Perspective on Codependency* (LifeWay Press, ISBN 0-8054-9973-3) or *Conquering Codependency: A Christ-Centered 12-Step Process* (LifeWay Press, ISBN 0-8054-9975-X).

Codependency

Codependents are addicted to persons or relationships rather than substances. They are characterized by caretaking behaviors such as feeling responsible for others and feeling compelled to help solve problems or fix feelings. They feel safest when giving, but are often angry when their help isn't effective or well-received.

Codependents say yes when they want to say no, do more than their fair share of work, and do things others are capable of doing for themselves. They try to please others rather than themselves. They are attracted to needy people and feel bored or worthless when they don't have a crisis, a problem to solve, or someone to help.

PERFECTIONISM

Perfectionism is easier to describe than to define. These symptoms were defined by David Seamands and Beth Funk in *Healing for Damaged Emotions Workbook:*[2]

- Tyranny of the oughts. Perfectionists live with "I ought to do better," "I ought to have done better," and "I ought to be able to do better."
- Self-depreciation. They're never good enough; God is never pleased with them.
- Anxiety. Their oversensitive consciences casts a cloud of guilt and anxiety.
- Legalism. They overemphasize externals, do's/don'ts, rules, and regulations.
- Anger. The perfectionist develops resentment against the oughts, the Christian faith, other Christians, himself, but saddest of all, against God.
- Denial. Seamands says, "Under the stress and the strain of trying to live with a self he can't like, a God he can't love, and other people he can't get along with, the strain can become too much. … Denial becomes a way of life."[2]

 Read the contrasts between Perfectionism and Excellence. Place an X on the following scale to describe yourself.

Perfectionism	Vs.	Excellence
Idealistic—how it should be		Realistic—how they are
Product-minded— I'll be happy when…		Process-minded—joy in the journey It is all process.
Sets impossible goals		Sets doable goals—can be done now!
Must be the best		Your best is all God wants.
Worth = Performance		Worth = God made you in His image.[3]

WELCOME DESPERATION

Two strategies can help us with the challenges of dark emotions, addictive behaviors and codependency, and perfectionism. The first of these, desperation, is cited as the first step in recovery programs. We must admit that our challenges are bigger than our willpower and ability to "fix."

For most of Tom's life he had avoided his feelings; he thought people who were touchy-feely were weak. Yet now Tom was pummeled by all sorts of emotions. He barely recovered from one assault when another rolled over him. It started the day he got word that his mother had cancer. At first he contained the long-stuffed emotions, but day 3 brought an open floodgate of feelings. Tom felt desperate for a solution! Desperation can leave you feeling hopeless. You look at what is facing you and want to shout, *It is too much!* This type of despair can lead to deep physiological fatigue and lethargy. Your emotions may be extremely raw and tender. You may feel that one more thing happening may break you into pieces. Desperation impacts body, mind, emotions, and spirit.

From God's viewpoint, desperation creates an opportunity to need Him in a way that a person never has before. The desperation stretches a person's soul, broadening the capacity to trust our Heavenly Father. It invites us to know God—not just know about Him. We see how desperation works in Mark 5:25-34. For 12 years the woman with the flow of blood had no relief, although she had done everything within her power to remedy the situation. She had emptied her financial resources with no improvement. Her situation was desperate.

 Perhaps you are facing a desperate situation. If so, write about it in the margin. If not, write a prayer for someone who faces such a situation.

This woman with the flow of blood heard about Jesus and decided to turn to Him. Luke's account of this story records that she "came from behind and touched the border of His garment. And immediately her flow of blood stopped" (Luke 8:44, NKJV). Her desperation and despair had driven her to the Source of life. She was well! What an experience! Her problem was gone, and she was whole again.

Suddenly Jesus stopped and asked, " 'Who touched me?' " (v. 45). He realized that a power surge had left His body. Peter's response is both comical and understandable: *Of course you have been touched. Look at the people pressing in on every side.* Peter did not understand that Jesus knows the difference between those who want to see, observe, or be entertained and those who turn to Him with a desperate faith.

What can we learn from this story? Here are a few of my ideas.
1. Everyone will encounter life difficulties that can lead to a sense of emotional desperation. God designed life in such a way that nothing truly satisfies our hearts but Him. You were designed to be fulfilled by Him alone.
2. What can you do with the emotional sense of desperation? You can feel utter hopelessness that leads to despair. You can cover the desperation of your heart with other forms of escape, or you can turn to Jesus.
3. Jesus knows those who want to use Him for their own selfish ends and those who truly want to touch Him—who must have Him. You cannot do anything that disqualifies you from an intimate relationship with Jesus. Nothing can separate you from His love and care (see Rom. 8:38-39).

Our Heavenly Father is pleased when our desperation turns into active faith. He longs to hear us ask for help. As God's children we can enter His royal throne room, a place where only the king's intimates may come, and say, *Dad, I need help!*—to which He responds with mercy. Remember the phrase, "I can't!"? (See p. 56.) This phrase allows us to admit our neediness and turn to God.

UPREACH

Read Psalm 139:1-3.
God sees our inner parts.
There is no secret with God.
Allow Him to search you
(v. 23-24) in order to bring
healing and wholeness
to your life.

"Let us therefore come boldly to the throne of grace, that we may obtain mercy and find grace to help in time of need."
—Hebrews 4:16, NKJV

PRACTICE "CRYING OUT" TO GOD

The emotional pressure had built for a couple of weeks, and I felt I was at the breaking point. I went upstairs to our unfinished attic and knelt in front of an old boxing bag laid long-ways on the floor. With all my might I hit the bag with both hands as I cried out to God for help. At first the emotions ran like white water on a rushing river. Then slowly they began to calm. I was in the attic probably an hour or so. Something happened that began to free me from dark, painful emotions.

After this, God taught me the importance of "crying out" to Him. In Psalms 30:2 the psalmist said, "O Lord my God, I cried out to You, and You healed me" (NKJV). As I read this, I thought, *That is what I experienced!*

Individuals experiencing high levels of pain literally "cry out" uncontrollably or yell at the top of their lungs. Some refer to this as a *catharsis*—a release of tension or a purging of emotions. The psalmist found an avenue to emotional health by simply expressing to God what he was experiencing. "Crying out to God" has become a major source of emotional growth and personal healing for me. I would like to offer you some of my own insights on the use of "crying out."

1. God is a realist! Often people tell God how they *should* live rather than how they *do* live. We have no need to hide anything from our gracious Father. He can handle whatever we bring to Him. We must "tell it like it is."
2. God is available even in our messes. I believed that God was only willing to help when I was living perfectly. As a result, I was unable to go to God when life was a mess—and for me that was most of the time. For "crying out" to work, I had to be able to view God as available no matter what my situation.
3. Don't give up. "Crying out" is not a quick fix; it is more about a living communion with God. Although some relief comes from the process of "crying out," healing and growth are the results of intimacy with God. As "crying out" reflects our relationship to Him, growth and health will occur.

In this chapter, we have examined several emotional challenges that can sidetrack your wellness journey. If you found yourself identifying with any of these to the point that your normal, daily routine is affected by it, consider these actions:

1. If a book was suggested, find it and begin reading. Talk to your pastor, church staff member, or another church leader about offering this study.
2. Ask your pastor, church staff member, or another church leader for the names of Christian counselors in your area. If you are looking for a counselor with specialized training in a certain area, mention that when you call or ask the referral sources for that information.
3. Call your physician and schedule a check-up as soon as possible. Chemical imbalances, mineral deficiencies, diabetes, and other health problems often reveal themselves through emotional symptoms.

INREACH

Do not ignore emotional challenges. They do not tend to improve with time. Seek help from God and others. He wants to guide you every step of your wellness journey.

---

[1]Dallas Willard, *The Divine Conspiracy* (San Francisco: HarperSanFrancisco, 1998), 148-149.
[2]David Seamands and Beth Funk, *Healing for Damaged Emotions Workbook* (Wheaton, Ill.: Victor Books, 1992), 107.
[3]Presented by Chris Thurmon at a meeting of the American Association of Christian Counselors in Kansas City, September 1998.

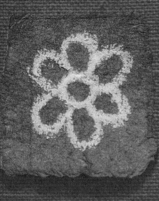

Week Ten

Your Emotional Wellness Journey

This study does not provide simple spiritual recipes that result in your never again facing troublesome emotions. Such recipes are fine for a casserole, but emotional wellness requires a vital, living relationship with Jesus Christ.

Television sitcoms solve problems quickly and easily, and magazines promise simple, effortless change. Change, however, is complex. It is not just difficult; we are incapable of meaningful and lasting change and growth apart from God. Rather than working intensely to quickly solve problems, we can persevere knowing that they are part of our growing into full stature in Christ.

Instead of a plan, we have a marvelous, magnificent, brilliant Father who loves us. Everyday events are soil for our growth. So let's rejoice, knowing that our God is able to complete the good work He has begun in us (Phil. 1:6).

In this final week, I want to share with you my emotional wellness journey and encourage you in your journey as well.

MY JOURNEY TOWARD EMOTIONAL WELLNESS

I returned home from taking our children to school and was speaking to my wife, Terri. I felt uneasy and anxious. Then something broke in me. I fell to the floor, my mind confused, my emotions uncontrollable. Tears and deep groans poured forth as I lay there, overwhelmed by this unknown enemy. It was as if something was choking the life out of me. Never had I known such internal pain. My introduction to emotional and spiritual brokenness stayed with me for almost two years.

The Crash

I call that morning in 1994 "the crash." Emotionally, spiritually, mentally, and physically. I fell apart! Soon I was diagnosed with severe clinical depression and required medication and in-depth psychiatric therapy for two years. I felt shame because I was a counseling professor at a seminary. If anyone should have known how to make life work, I should have. Obviously, I did not. Unknown to me, God was at work. I had started on an unusual, abrupt, and painful journey of healing.

INREACH

We have identified *busyness* as an enemy of emotional wellness. Have you taken steps to incorporate more stillness and solitude into your lifestyle? (See pages 53-54.)

Somewhere along the journey, God communicated to me that being weak and broken is OK. In fact, it is essential to knowing deep, abiding trust in Him!

Several things contributed to my crash. **First**, I ignored all human limits (especially emotional), pushing to do increasingly more until my body broke. I had no idea I was overloaded. When I felt tired, fearful, anxious, or overwhelmed, I assumed something was wrong with me. I believed I was responsible for *everyone* and *everything!* **Second**, I felt I was not good enough. I could never meet my own standards and covered this gnawing emotion by acting OK. In other words, I faked it. I had a major disconnection between who I was on the inside and how I presented myself. The only way I knew to quieten the condemning voice inside was busyness and achievement. I was constantly running, yet getting nowhere.

After a while I had no identity apart from the busyness and activity. I was no longer able to separate who I was from what I did. One problem with this performance mentality was that my performance always could have been better. Mike Yaconelli, co-founder of Youth Specialities, says this about the trap of performance, "I knew I was a sinner. I knew I continually disappointed God, but I could never accept that part of me. It was a part of me that embarrassed me. I continually felt the need to apologize, to run from my weaknesses, to deny who I was and concentrate on what I should be. I was broken, yes, but I was continually trying never to be broken again."[1] Like Mike, I was trying to hide my brokenness in unending activity. The emotional result was suffocating shame. Emotionally, there seemed no way out.

Third, I viewed God as always dissatisfied with me. Whenever I went to Him in prayer, I imagined a frown on His face. I just knew God was thinking, *You are such a disappointment to Me. Can't you do any better than that?* I would hang my head and mentally walk away, determined in my heart never to fail Him again. I would promise God never to be angry again, only to fall right back into the same pattern. During times of failure, I could not conceive of God running to help me. I only pictured His watching me fail—with no compassion or concern, just disdain and disgust.

This view of God resulted in significant emotional pain and confusion. I believed I deserved every bad thing that happened to me. It made perfect sense to me that God would not want to help someone so useless. Why would Someone as magnificent and marvelous as God truly concern Himself with the likes of me? When the crash occurred, I knew it was my fault, and I deserved everything I got.

Weakness Embraced

Despair was destroying me. Months of insomnia and anxiety sapped all my energy. Unsure whether I would be able to teach, fears wracked me. Would I lose my job? How would we pay bills? Would this damage my children? Could my wife endure my being emotionally and spiritually incapacitated? Would I ever get better?

Somewhere along the journey, God communicated to me that being weak and broken is OK. In fact, it is essential to knowing deep, abiding trust in Him! I could not believe that being weak and broken had any value, yet that is exactly what the Lord was teaching me. The crash was the vehicle that He used to instruct me in the way of weakness. I must confess, I was a slow learner.

Gradually, God's truth began to sink in. As I read His Word, passages such as 2 Corinthians 12:9 (NKJV) had new meaning. God said to Paul, "My strength is made perfect in weakness." Those simple words reached deep inside me and persuaded my heart that admitting weakness is central to a rich, growing relationship with Christ. Something in me was freed as Christ ministered this truth to my heart. I no longer had to be *strong*. I only had to rest in the One who is all-powerful, whose arms never fail, and whose strength is sufficient for all I will ever face.

Listen to Mike Yaconelli, who also found the path of weakness to be his source of strength: "I had totally misunderstood the Christian faith. I came to see that it was in my brokenness, in my powerlessness, in my weakness that Jesus was made strong. It was in the acceptance of my lack of faith that God could give me faith. It was in the embracing of my brokenness that I could identify with others' brokenness."[2]

 Read in the margin some Scriptures that were important to my growth and understanding. As you read them, underline the words that communicate the truths I was learning about the Christian faith.

God used Matthew 9:9-13 mightily in my life. Jesus called Matthew (a reject like me) to follow Him. The religious leaders were displeased with Jesus' being with and wanting to use people such as Matthew. Jesus said to them, " 'Those who are well have no need of a physician, but those who are sick' " (9:12, NKJV). Jesus knew all of us need a physician; all are in need of a Savior. Admitting sickness and neediness draws the Great Physician to us. We *all* need Him, must have Him, can't exist without Him. We were designed to be totally dependent on Him—alone.

I was getting it! Ever so slowly my heart was being renewed by admitting to God who I really was: one who could do nothing apart from Him. I believe He had waited a long time to hear those words from me.

I Learned to Cry Out to God

Before I fully grasped the reality of God as Father, I was so desperate that all I knew to do was to cry out to God. I would turn on the bathroom fan (so no one would hear), get in the shower, and cry out to God in overwhelming brokenness. It sounded like, "God, You are killing me! I don't think I can take any more! If I don't get relief soon, I am not going to make it." The heavens seemed deafeningly silent. I felt alone, abandoned by the only One who could help. Hopelessness turned to despair. I was learning a difficult emotional and spiritual lesson—that I had to distrust myself to be able to trust God.

The words of Proverbs 3:5 came to mind: "lean not on your own understanding." All my life I had leaned on my own understanding. I survived difficulties by leaning on myself since I did not seem to have anyone else. I was the protector and provider of my soul. As of September, 1994, I was unable to fulfill that role, motivating me to "cry out," but the lessons did not stop there. Part of being my Father's child was continually "crying out" to an attentive and concerned Heavenly Father. I could tell Him all, not just the good. He wanted all of me, not just what I deemed acceptable.

"The sacrifices of God are a broken spirit;
a broken and contrite heart,
O God, you will not despise."
—Psalm 51:17

" 'I am the vine; you are the branches. If a man remains in me and I in him, he will bear much fruit; apart from me you can do nothing.' "
—John 15:5

"Not that we are competent in ourselves to claim anything for ourselves, but our competence comes from God."
—2 Corinthians 3:5

"Let us then approach the throne of grace with confidence, so that we may receive mercy and find grace to help us in our time of need."
—Hebrews 4:16

"Trust in the Lord with all your heart
and lean not on your own understanding;
in all your ways acknowledge him,
and he will make your paths straight."
—Proverbs 3:5-6

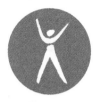

UPREACH

Go ahead. Try it. Cry out to God. Tell Him whatever is troubling you. Perhaps my method of releasing pent-up emotions to the Great Physician will work for you as well.

I began telling Him about my temptations. This was new to me; I had fought with all my might rather than to "cry out" to the One who could sustain and deliver me. Now I went to Him constantly—and you can too! His ears are attentive to our cries.

God as "Abba"

Before the crash, I feared that God was not good or loving—that somehow He did not care about me. This view added to my self-hate. I concur with Brennan Manning in his book, *Abba's Child:* "Self-hatred is the dominant malaise crippling Christians, and stifling their growth in the Holy Spirit."[3] I was crippled, but I soon learned God loves the crippled. Part of my emotional healing and growth was more clearly understanding who God is.

God knew I must rid myself of false ideas about Him. He showed me He was more loving than I could imagine. Ephesians 3:19 (NKJV) speaks of the "love of Christ which passes knowledge," a love greater than the mind can grasp. How can I tell you what this realization did for my love-sick heart? He loves me! He really loves me!

Dallas Willard says, "The acid test of *any* theology is this: Is the God presented one that can be loved, heart, soul, mind, and strength? If the thoughtful, honest answer is; 'Not really,' then we need to look elsewhere or deeper. It does not really matter how sophisticated intellectually or doctrinally our approach is. If it fails to set a *lovable* God—radiant, happy, friendly, accessible, and totally competent being—before ordinary people, we have gone wrong."[4] One key aspect was seeing God as *Abba* (Aramaic word for *father* or *daddy).*

My father died one month before my emotional breakdown. His death was a major contributor to my collapse, triggering many painful memories. Our family had our share of problems, but I had taken an ostrich's approach—if I did not look at them, maybe they would go away. Dad's death opened the door to many painful aspects of my past that I could no longer hold in check. Little did I know the Master would use these memories to draw me nearer.

After Dad's death, an image came to me: I crawled up on Dad's lap; he embraced me and said, *It's going to be OK.* Even though Dad had hurt me, this image was branded on my mind. I could not get rid of it. Amidst the pain of this loss, God began to teach me He is my Abba; my Father; my Daddy. He directed me to Romans 8:15 (NKJV), "You did not receive the spirit of bondage again to fear, but you received the Spirit of adoption by whom we cry out, 'Abba, Father.' " The thought of God as Father took on new meaning. I would never lose my Heavenly Dad. He'd never leave or forsake me. I knew it in my head; now it was coming to life in my heart. The *in my heart* part was new to me. It is beyond intellect. It is the assurance of a heart that knows the Father's love and embrace.

I felt like the prodigal son in Luke 15. Although I had not committed rank overt sin, I knew I was unworthy and undeserving of the Father's love. I felt shame about who I was rather than guilt over what I had done. The results were the same: both the prodigal and I "knew" we could never be accepted as a son.

As I read the familiar parable, I was shocked at the father's response, " 'While he was still a long way off, his father saw him and was filled with compassion for him; he ran to his son, threw his arms around him and kissed him' " (v. 20). It was too good to be true. Had I been the father, I would have run out, shaken my accusing finger in his face, and told him how horrible he had been. But the father in the parable did the opposite. He had compassion and embraced his son. As I searched my memories, I could not remember anyone being that bad and being treated that well. This action was not human—it was God!

For the first time, not only did I feel the Heavenly Father's embrace, but I received His embrace. Normally, I would have pulled away, feeling that I was undeserving. Yet I collapsed in His arms, my heart overwhelmed with His acceptance. I knew He would never let me go. I no longer believed I was an imposition to God; now I fully believed that He enjoyed me (Zeph. 3:16-17). No longer enslaved to guilt, shame, self-hate, discouragement, performance, or fear, I was a son! I knew Him affectionately as "Abba."

 Are you comfortable picturing yourself in God the Father's lap? What feelings does this image convey to you? Write them in the margin.

Intimacy With Others

In my darkness intimate friends were a necessity—mine were four male soul mates and my wife, Terri. They were anchors for me during my transition from self- to Christ-life. Let me explain their role in a story. The crash was a raging river that was beating me to death. I was at the mercy of the current, my life jacket shredded by the velocity of the river. I was doomed. Suddenly ten hands firmly grasped me. I was no longer drowning; they had jumped in with me. I can't emphasize enough the importance of their getting in the midst of the problem with me. Each was wearing a life jacket; they kept me afloat. Hope surged through my being. Their presence reactivated my faith. I began to believe I might make it.

Their words were most important. As they held onto me, they said things like, "We are with you, Paul," "You can depend on us to stick it out with you," "We don't have answers, but we offer ourselves to you," and "We will continue to trust in the Heavenly Father until your faith grows." They did not try to fix me—there was *no* fix. God gave me Himself and friends, not a formula.

Our gracious Heavenly Father provided me with courageous soul mates who entered the treacherous waters of my life, not sure of anything except their love for God and for me. Gradually, they loosened their grip on me as I began to understand how to allow Abba to be my life jacket. The urgent need for them subsided, and we returned to a more normal Christian intimacy.

My Emotional Growth Continues

Several years later, I continue to grow. Growth is not so much a destination to reach as it is a relationship with God to develop. I encourage you to continue in the wellness journey. Emotional growth and maturity really do happen! May my

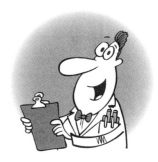

Professor Phitt says:
The prodigal son's father was able to run to his son (who was still a long way off) to welcome him home. Would you have been able to welcome the prodigal in this manner? Or would he have had to come to you? Explain your answer.

OUTREACH

We must have others to
help us bear our burdens, and
we must be willing and ready
to assist others when their
lives turn into raging rivers.
If you have been such a friend,
thank you. If you need such a
friend, ask the Father to
supply your need.

Wellness is achieved
one wise choice at a time.

life be a testimony to you. In times of desperation and difficulty, remember that you are not the only one who has been on this path. I and many others have gone before. Hold tight to Abba's hand and never forget His heart is full of love for you.

YOUR EMOTIONAL WELLNESS JOURNEY

Now that we have looked at my emotional-wellness journey, take a few moments to reflect on your own journey. Perhaps yours has not been as tumultuous as mine. I hope not. You may have grown up in a more emotionally healthy environment, or you may have had a more complete picture of God.

Others of you can identity with my journey. Perhaps you are still in the midst of the storm. Hopefully, your outcome will bring to you as much joy as mine has brought to me. If you are past the storm, join me in praising our loving Abba Father for all He has brought you through.

Look again at the goals you set during week 2 (p. 24). Which of these words represent your feelings about your progress? (Circle all that apply.)

satisfied   encouraged   dissatisfied   discouraged

Review the change process (pp. 63-64). Fill in the chart below to reflect what you feel still needs to happen for you to reach your goals:

Awareness _____

Knowledge_____

Action _____

Change _____

A JOURNEY ... NOT A DESTINATION

Wherever you find yourself today, remember that all of us have a lifetime of baggage to unload and a future of continuing to grow in our relationship to God, to ourselves, and to each other. Continue to use the stress model on page 13 and the feelings chart on page 48. Refer to the change process on pages 63-64. This study represents a lifetime of learning for me, and you, too, will continue to learn valuable lessons in emotional wellness. You are on a journey. Arriving is not as important as the process by which you get there. Wellness is achieved one wise choice at a time.

[1]Brennan Manning, *Abba's Child* (Colorado Springs: NavPress, 1994), 52.
[2]Ibid.
[3]Ibid., 20.
[4]Dallas Willard, *The Divine Conspiracy* (San Francisco: HarperSanFrancisco, 1998), 329.

How to Become a Christian

We were created as emotional beings capable of giving and receiving love. One of the greatest feelings we have on this earth is loving and being loved by someone else. God wants us to love Him above anyone or anything else because loving Him puts everything else in life in perspective. In Him, we find the hope, peace, and joy that is only possible through a personal relationship with God. Through His presence in our lives, we can truly love others, because God is love. Love comes from God (1 John 4:7-8).

John 3:16 says, "God so loved the world that he gave his one and only Son, that whoever believes in him shall not perish but have eternal life." In order to live our earthly lives "to the full" (see John 10:10), we must accept God's gift of love.

A relationship with God begins by admitting that we are not perfect and continue to fall short of God's standards. Romans 3:23 says, "All have sinned and fall short of the glory of God." The price for these wrongdoings is separation from God. We deserve to pay the price for our sin. "The wages (or price) of sin is death, but the gift of God is eternal life in Christ Jesus our Lord" (Rom. 6:23).

God's love comes to us right in the middle of our sin. "But God demonstrates his own love for us in this: While we were still sinners, Christ died for us" (Rom. 5:8). He doesn't ask us to clean up our lives first—in fact, without His help, we are incapable of living by His standards. He wants us to come to Him as we are.

Forgiveness begins when we admit our sin to God. When we do, He is faithful to forgive and restore our relationship with Him. "If we confess our sins, he is faithful and just and will forgive us our sins and purify us from all unrighteousness" (1 John 1:9).

Scripture confirms that this love gift and relationship with God is not just for a special few, but for everyone. "Everyone who calls on the name of the Lord will be saved" (Romans 10:13).

If you would like to receive God's gift of salvation, pray this prayer:

> Dear God, I know that I am imperfect and separated from You. Please forgive me of my sin and adopt me as Your child. Thank You for this gift of life through the sacrifice of Your Son. I will live my life for You. Amen.

If you prayed this prayer for the first time, you are now a child of God. In your Bible, read 1 John 5:11-12. This verse assures you that if you have accepted God's Son, Jesus Christ, as your Savior and Lord, you have this eternal life.

Share your experience with your *Fit 4* facilitator, someone in your group, your pastor, or a trusted Christian friend. Welcome to God's family!

Leader Guide

With All My Heart: God's Design for Emotional Wellness is a continuing study in *Fit 4: A LifeWay Christian Wellness Plan.* This study is open to anyone who chooses to participate, whether or not the person has taken another *Fit 4* course or continuing study. Treat it as you would any one-hour group discipleship course.

Relationship to *Fit 4*
Review pages 4 and 5 to understand how this study incorporates the basic principles of *Fit 4.*

Because this study emphasizes only one of four essential components of wellness, encourage participants to use the *Accountability Journal* provided with each *Member Book* to record daily food and exercise choices. Some participants may not have committed to the *Fit 4 Guidelines for Healthy Eating* (see *Journal,* p. 20) or the *Fit 4* F.I.T.T. exercise model for developing a personalized exercise plan (see *Journal,* p. 14). Promote the concept of whole-person health by encouraging nutritional and fitness goals as an integral part of total wellness. The Professor Phitt suggestions each week offer practical application activities.

Introductory Session
Because of the *Fit 4* terminology used, as well as references to Professor Phitt and other *Fit 4* resources, we recommend that participants view the 15-minute *Fit 4* Introductory Session video found at the beginning of both the *Fitness* and *Nutrition* group session videos in the *Fit 4 Plan Kit* (ISBN 0-6330-0580-0). Preview the video and have it cued at the beginning of the tape. Arrange for a TV/VCR for the introductory session only. A lesson plan for the introductory session is found on page 89.

Sessions 1-10
Each week's reading assignment in the *Member Book* can be read in one sitting or spaced throughout the week. Encourage participants to memorize the Verse(s) to Know and say the Scripture together at the beginning of each session. Session plans for the 10 weeks are found on pages 89-94. They are guides to help you lead discussion.

Encourage participants to ask questions and make comments from their reading. The benefit to each participant will increase as he or she completes each lesson's margin

Lifestyle Discipline activities as well as the learning activities highlighted by the *Fit 4* logo. Calling attention to these elements of the lesson will promote their use. Otherwise, members may assume they are unimportant.

Leading the Wrap-Up Session
Session 11 (week 12 of the study) is the final session of each *Fit 4* continuing course. In this session, lead a time of sharing, reflection, planning for the future, and praying. Several ideas for informal closure activities are suggested on page 94. Review these a few weeks before session 11 so you can plan ahead. Include the class in the planning.

Your Role as Facilitator
Like other members of your group, you are on your own wellness journey. No one is looking to you as an expert on emotional wellness. Your role is to guide the group experience using the session plans provided.

Before each session, arrive early. Place chairs in a circle and sit with other members. Provide a sign-up sheet at the door and name tags, if needed. Have on hand extra Bibles, pens or pencils, and *Member Books* for the first two sessions. Pray for each member, the group process, and yourself on a regular basis. Use the attendance sheet to note absentees; then call them during the week.

Begin and end each session on time. Open and close the sessions with prayer. Encourage member discussion of the week's material. Avoid doing too much talking. Keep the discussion positive, in keeping with the emphasis on emotional wellness. Avoid letting members get too personal or graphic in sharing.

Be aware of special needs in the class. If a class member is unsaved, be prepared to follow the leadership of the Holy Spirit to know the right time to talk to that person privately to lead them to Christ (see How to Become a Christian, p. 87). If other problems surface, be prepared to refer members to Christian counselors in the area.

After the session, complete your weekly reading assignment and your *Accountability Journal.* Learn each week's Verse(s) to Know. Follow the instructions in this Guide for planning for the next session.

INTRODUCTORY SESSION

Session Goals

To introduce participants to the concept of whole-person health based on Mark 12:30-31 and to enlist participation in this study.

Before the Session

- Set up the TV/VCR and cue the tape to the Introductory Session video.
- Arrange chairs so everyone can see the TV screen and each other.
- Supply name tags for each person.
- Provide an attendance sheet and pen.
- Have on hand one copy of the *Member Book* and *Accountability Journal* for every person expected.
- Before members arrive, pray for God's guidance.

During the Session

Greet members as they arrive. Have them sign the attendance sheet and give a phone number or email address. Instruct them to complete and wear the provided name tag. Open with prayer.

Introduce yourself and ask participants to share their names and one interesting fact about themselves. Distribute copies of *With All My Heart: God's Design for Emotional Wellness* and the *Accountability Journal*.

Explain that although this study is open to anyone, it is a continuing study in *Fit 4: A LifeWay Christian Wellness Plan*. Say: *During this session we will watch the* **Fit 4** *Introductory Session video to acquaint you with the concept of whole-person health and to introduce you to terms that will be used throughout the study.* Ask members to turn to page 6 in their *Member Books* and write responses on the Viewer Guide as you play the Introductory Session video.

Ask volunteers to share responses to the Viewer Guide. Review pages 4 and 5 of the *Member Book*. Then ask participants to put together their *Accountability Journals*. Highlight the information on pages 4-25. Explain that the *Accountability Journal* is a voluntary tool to encourage a wellness lifestyle. No one will evaluate their entries. Ask them to turn to page 26, circle tomorrow's day, and write the date. Encourage the group to begin tomorrow recording their food and exercise choices.

Overview week 1 in their *Member Books*. Explain the purpose of the Verse to Know and the margin activities. Point out that the material can be read in one sitting or by sections throughout the week. Call attention to page 95, which lists other **Fit 4** resources, such as the *fit4.com* Web site and the *Christian Health* magazine.

Allow time for participants to ask questions. Collect payment for materials, if needed. Close the session with a word of encouragement and prayer.

SESSION 1

Session Goals

To understand how emotions relate to our physical bodies, minds, and spirits. To appreciate the importance of emotional wellness in whole-person health.

During the Session

As members arrive, ask them to sign the attendance sheet and wear a name tag (optional). Allow 2-3 minutes for prayer requests and enlist a volunteer to pray.

Say or read together the Verses to Know (p. 7). Ask someone to recall the example of the chest of drawers from the opening paragraphs of week 1.

Review key points from each of the major headings by asking questions such as: *How are emotions physical, spiritual, mental, relational? How do they add value and meaning to our lives?* Emphasize specific statements you may have underlined as you read.

Ask members to turn to the stress model on page 13. Form two or more teams; ask each to illustrate the stress model with a real or made-up event/stressor and follow it through the model. After 5-7 minutes, call for reports.

Enlist volunteers to share their responses to the **UPREACH, OUTREACH,** and **INREACH** activities in the margin. Share responses to the last activity on page 12. Ask if anyone followed Professor Phitt's advice about a walking program. Share responses to the last activity on page 14.

Overview session 2, creating interest in the topic. Conclude the session by reading together the closing prayer on page 14.

SESSION 2

Session Goals

To affirm that we are emotional beings created in God's image. To identify the purpose for this study.

During the Session

Greet members and have them sign the attendance sheet. Call for prayer requests and enlist a volunteer to pray. Say or read together the Verse to Know (p. 15). Brainstorm possible meanings of being made in the image of God (see p. 20).

Ask: *Did it surprise you that God is an emotional Being? Why or why not?* After several responses, ask: *How are God's expressions of these emotions different from our own: (1) anger; (2) jealousy.*

Invite reactions to this statement from page 20: "God could have struck from the record any reference to anger or sadness, but He chose to leave it for us to read today." Summarize by saying that God's emotional expressions encourage us to feel and express our emotions, even those we label as dark emotions.

Ask: *Do you find it surprising that great leaders of the Bible experienced dark emotions? Why or why not?* Then ask: *What can we learn from reading about their emotional expressions?*

Emphasize the purpose of this study from page 23. Encourage members to seek God's plan for emotional wellness rather than the latest self-help or popular psychology approach. Say: *When we seek God, He will reveal Himself to us.* Ask members to turn to Jeremiah 24:7 and enlist a volunteer to read the verse aloud.

Allow a few minutes for members to review or complete the goals for this study (p. 24). If your group is comfortable with each other, invite volunteers to share one or more of their goals. Or form pairs or groups of three and have each small group discuss their goals.

If you have used small groups, reconvene the large group. Overview week 3 and read the Verse to Know. Close with prayer, thanking God for making us in His image as emotional creatures. Thank Him for His plan for emotional wellness.

SESSION 3

Session Goals

To identify ways each of the six factors in emotional development contributes to or detracts from emotional wellness. To review the plan of salvation.

During the Session

Greet members and have them sign the attendance sheet. Call for prayer requests and enlist a volunteer to pray. Say or read together the Verse to Know (p. 25). Invite several responses to the question, *What does it mean to seek God with all your heart?*

Review the Professor Phitt suggestion from page 25. Allow members to comment on their experiences in keeping the *Accountability Journal*. Answer questions and provide encouragement.

Assign one of the six factors in emotional development to individuals, pairs, or groups of three or more. Make this assignment: (1) How does this factor contribute to emotional wellness? (2) How can this factor detract from emotional wellness? When the majority of the members have completed the assignment, call for the six reports.

Invite responses to the activity at the top of page 34. Have respondents share their personality combination and emotions they feel are common to this style. Members may disagree with each other. Allow for differences and affirm each individual's uniqueness.

Remind the group that one of the purposes of this study is to learn to respond emotionally in ways that enhance our relationships with God, others, and ourselves. Invite responses to this statement from page 34: "The degree to which your emotional past dictates your choices today is just that: your choice."

Ask members to turn in their Bibles to Ephesians 4:22-32 and enlist a volunteer to read the verses aloud. Ask: *What is the "new self"? What are characteristics of the new self?* Review page 87, which explains how we receive this new self. Ask if anyone prayed the prayer to accept Christ. Offer to talk with the person(s) after the session. Close with prayer that members will grow in putting on the new self through Christ.

SESSION 4

Session Goal

To point to our relationship with God as the true Source of belonging, worth, and competence.

During the Session

Greet members and have them sign the attendance sheet. Call for prayer requests and enlist a volunteer to pray. Say or read together the Verse to Know (p. 35).

Display a large sheet of paper that you have divided into three columns labeled "Belonging," "Worth," and "Competence" (building blocks). Down the left side space out the words "Presence," "Absence," and "Cultivate."

Brainstorm answers to these questions for each of the three building blocks: *How do we demonstrate the presence of this building block? How do we demonstrate the absence of this building block? How do we cultivate this building block in our lives?* Ask a volunteer to write responses on the chart under the appropriate heading.

As the group shares information for "Belonging," encourage the actions suggested in the OUTREACH activity (p. 35). For "Worth," invite responses to the INREACH activity (p. 38). For "Competence," discuss the answer to the UPREACH activity (p. 39).

Invite responses to the first activity on page 40 by asking volunteers to share a time when they experienced each of these building-block feelings and/or to share a time when they experienced the lack of each of these feelings. You may need to model the role by sharing your own experiences. Ask volunteers only to respond.

Ask members to turn to Galatians 4:4-7 in their Bibles and enlist a volunteer to read the verses aloud. Emphasize that our belonging, worth, and competence are based on our position in Christ: we are sons and heirs. Our relationship with God allows us to come to Him as a loving Father, who graciously gives us all we need to accomplish His purposes for our lives.

Invite sentence prayers, thanking God for His acceptance, forgiveness, and love.

SESSION 5

Session Goal

To encourage self understanding and understanding of others through improving speaking and listening skills.

During the Session

Greet members and have them sign the attendance sheet. Call for prayer requests and enlist a volunteer to pray.

Lead members to recall the five components of emotional wellness. Ask: *Why do you think the author began with the first and fourth components? Why don't we better understand our own emotions and the emotions of others?*

Say or read together the Verses to Know (p. 41). Point out that only God can remove the blinders of sin. Ask members to turn in their Bibles to John 12:40 and 2 Corinthians 4:4-6. Enlist volunteers to read the passages aloud. Emphasize Christ as the Source of light.

Call for several responses to the question on page 43, "How would becoming more emotionally literate affect your life?" Then ask members to turn to the feelings chart on page 48. Assign each face to a volunteer. Ask each volunteer to make the face and explain the feeling, using as many feeling words as possible. Encourage the use of this chart as the study continues.

Ask: *How can identifying historical emotions help us express our emotions in more appropriate ways?* (p. 43-44). Invite volunteers to give examples of each of the four suggestions for sharing emotions (pp. 44-45).

Ask: *Why is empathy difficult for us? Why is empathy essential to building relationship skills?* Invite responses to the OUTREACH activity on page 46.

Optional activity: Lead the group to role-play some examples of ineffective and effective listening by assigning pairs to create and perform a short dialogue. Ask listeners to identify the listening principle that was illustrated or violated.

Call attention to the suggestion by Professor Phitt on page 47. Encourage exercise as a proper way to recharge our emotional batteries. Close with prayer.

SESSION 6

Session Goal

To encourage practicing the five strategies that help us improve relationships by managing emotions in a healthy manner.

During the Session

Greet members and have them sign the attendance sheet. Call for prayer requests and enlist a volunteer to pray.

Ask members to turn to page 56 in their *Member Books* and locate the five strategies for managing emotions that they wrote in the margin. Beside each strategy, have them write a number between 1 and 5 to indicate the degree to which they practice this strategy (1 is infrequent and 5 is frequently). Do not ask for responses. Encourage members to apply all of these principles.

Review the strategies in one of two ways:
1. Review as a large group, asking these questions for each strategy:
   • What are advantages of applying this strategy?
   • What are disadvantages of not using this strategy?
   • What are some practical ways to begin using this strategy?
2. Assign each strategy to a pair or small group to review using the same questions. After 5-7 minutes for discussion, call for reports. Allow questions and comments from other groups after each report.

Say or read together the Verse to Know (p. 49). Emphasize that self-discipline is from God. Compare this Scripture with Galatians 5:22-23 (p. 51). Enlist a volunteer to read aloud 1 Peter 5:8-9. Say: *Self-control is a major factor in resisting temptation.*

Point out that in addition to practicing self-discipline in emotional expression, we are to practice self-discipline in our food and exercise choices. Review Professor Phitt's advice on page 55.

Invite responses to the OUTREACH activity on page 53 and the INREACH activity on page 55. Close with prayer, thanking God for His answers to prayer that reflect His love and care for us.

SESSION 7

Session Goals

To determine ways our minds, souls, and bodies contribute to emotional motivation. To be able to use emotional energy as positive motivators for life goals.

During the Session

Greet members and have them sign the attendance sheet. Call for prayer requests and enlist a volunteer to pray. Say or read together the Verse to Know. Ask: *What is the key to acting according to God's purposes?* (God)

Read the session goal. Have members review the stress model on page 13. Invite reactions to the statement, "Because we each have the ability to change our thoughts, we can change how we feel." As a group, discuss the activities on pages 58-59.

Make the transition to how our spiritual selves influence our emotions. As a group, discuss the activities on pages 60-61. Invite reactions to the margin quote on page 61. Ask: *How does your view of God affect your feelings?* Be sensitive to anyone in the group who seems to struggle with inaccurate views of God. Offer to meet with him or her outside class time, if possible.

Ask members to think of ways our bodies affect our feelings when we experience 1) sleep deprivation; 2) lack of exercise; 3) inadequate nutrition; or 4) stress. As a group, discuss the activity on page 63.

Ask members to locate Acts 10 in their Bibles. Use the story of Peter's vision to illustrate the change process (pp. 63-64). Then have them locate Galatians 2:11-14. Enlist a volunteer to read aloud these verses as an example of how imperfection does not need to discourage us.

Invite volunteers to share actions they have taken to lead them to specific life changes. Be prepared to share your own list as a discussion starter. Review Professor Phitt's advice on page 62. For more information on resistance training, consult pages 42-47 in *Fit 4* Fitness Member Workbook (see p. 95 for ordering information). Close with prayer that members' emotional energies will positively motivate them to accomplish God's plans for their lives.

SESSION 8

Session Goal

To encourage the development of relationship skills that enhance rather than stifle relationships.

During the Session

Greet members and have them sign the attendance sheet. Call for prayer requests and enlist a volunteer to pray. Say or read together the Verse to Know (p. 65). Ask: *What does it mean to love others?* After several responses, ask a volunteer to read aloud 1 Corinthians 13:4-7. Point out that love is a way of acting toward others more than it is a warm, fuzzy feeling. Summarize the importance of choosing to develop relationship skills as a sign of members' desire to grow in emotional maturity.

Optional activity: Assign pairs to role-play each of the habits that stifle relationships (pp. 65-66). Allow 3-5 minutes for pairs to make up dialogues that illustrates the habits. Then call for role-plays. If you do not use this activity, ask volunteers to illustrate ways each of the habits are displayed on a daily basis.

Review the three coping styles on page 67. Emphasize the healthy pattern of coping described on page 68 (risking emotional exposure by trusting God for protection and control). Point out that the more self-protective and guarded we are, the less likely we are to have authentic, open, and honest communication.

Review the five levels of communication (p. 69), asking volunteers to make up a sentence illustrating each one. Emphasize the importance of using levels 3 and 4 on a more consistent basis in order to develop more meaningful relationships.

Call attention to the OUTREACH activity on page 71. Ask a volunteer to read Proverbs 16:28 and 20:19. Remind members of the importance of confidentiality in building trust.

Enlist a volunteer to recall the story of Paul and Onesiphorus as an example of soul-mate relationships. Invite volunteers to tell about a soul-mate relationship.

As members bow in prayer, read aloud the prayer on page 72 or pray a prayer of your own.

SESSION 9

Session Goal

To identify appropriate actions to deal with challenges to emotional wellness.

During the Session

Because of the sensitive nature of this week's material, do not ask pointed questions or call for responses of a private, personal nature. If someone has identified an addictive behavior, for example, offer your assistance outside of class to pursue other avenues of help. Do not allow this session to become a counseling session. If possible, display on a table at the front of the room some or all of the resources listed in this chapter.

As the session begins, greet members and have them sign the attendance sheet. Call for prayer requests and enlist a volunteer to pray. Say or read together the Verse to Know (p. 73). Point out that God's peace is felt during the storms of life; peace is not the absence of storms.

Explain that everyone deals with dark emotions. Recall the statement from page 73: "No emotion should dominate or control us. When dark emotions continually envelope us, we should consider ourselves sidetracked on the journey to emotional wellness." Invite questions and discuss issues raised by members from pages 73-76, including the INREACH activity on page 74.

Emphasize the definition of addiction as dependence on something or someone other than God (p. 76). Ask: *Why are the following poor substitutes for God: drugs, alcohol, tobacco, food, and people or relationships (codependency)?* Discuss the OUTREACH activity on page 78. If persons in the group are struggling with addictive behaviors, recommend professional Christian counseling. Ask your church office for a list of Christian counselors in your area. Read the INREACH activity on page 80.

Review the characteristics of perfectionism and contrast it with a desire for excellence (p. 78). Discuss the two strategies for dealing with emotional challenges (welcome desperation and practice crying out to God).

Optional: Call attention to the resources on the display table. Close with prayer.

SESSION 10

Session Goals

To review the major ideas from this study. To share progress on the emotional wellness journey.

During the Session

This session serves as a review of the study and an opportunity for members to share their wellness journey. Adapt the lesson plan to reflect the personality of your group, their needs, and their interests.

As the session begins, lead the group to recall answers to prayer during the past 10 weeks. Spend time praising God for His faithfulness. Say or read together the Verse to Know (p. 81). Discuss the contrast between someone who exalts himself (self-centered, self-seeking) and someone who is humble (God-centered, seeks kingdom purposes). Ask members to locate in their Bibles Philippians 2:5-11, and enlist a volunteer to read the passage aloud. Summarize by saying that Jesus perfectly illustrates Matthew 23:12.

Walk members through every page of *With All My Heart*, pausing to discuss ideas members have underlined or found especially helpful. This process may take more than half of the session. Here are some discussion starters:

1. How does the stress model (p. 13) help you analyze how you react to events/stressors?
2. How does your emotional history affect your life today (week 3)?
3. What are the five components of emotional wellness?
4. How has your emotional vocabulary grown as a result of this study (p. 48)?

Enlist someone to review the author's emotional wellness journey, emphasizing what he learned about God, himself, and his relationships with others (pp. 81-85).

Optional activity: Ask members to share in pairs or threesomes their emotional wellness journeys—what they have learned about God, themselves, and their relationships with others. If your group would not be comfortable with this approach, share your own journey. Announce plans for next week's session. Encourage members to review the Verses to Know during the coming week. Close with prayer.

SESSION 11

Session Goals

To set goals to maintain progress in the emotional wellness journey. To provide closure for the group experience.

During the Session

Select an option below or determine your own closure activities with the group. Additional options can be found in the lesson plans for the *Fit 4* *Nutrition* and *Fitness* courses in the *Facilitator Guide* (see pp. 44 and 70).

Option 1:

Lead members to share what the group experience has meant to them. Provide materials such as construction paper, felt-tip markers, chenile craft stems, glue, and scissors. Instruct members to make a visual "thank you" for one or more members of the group. Make sure that no one is left out. Take turns making the presentations.

Select volunteers to review their goals from page 24 and their plans for future progress on page 86. Encourage members to continue using the *Accountability Journal* (ordering information on p. 95). Announce plans for the next *Fit 4* continuing study or other discipleship option.

Review the study's Verses to Know. Close with prayer and a personal word of encouragement.

Option 2:

Using an emotion-based story, discuss various emotions and situations based on what members have learned. The story could be a Bible story, a familiar novel, a children's book, or an appropriate movie. If you choose the movie, allow time to view the movie and discuss it. You may want to host this meeting in a home. Plan accordingly. Ask members for suggestions during the week.

Use comments and questions such as: Describe the various relationships in the story. What was the story's emotional range? What can we learn from the story about both positive and negative emotional reactions? Which character best describes your reaction to this type of situation? How would you respond the same or differently?

Lead the class in a time of commitment and close with a thanksgiving prayer.

FIT 4 RESOURCES

Fit 4 *Plan Kit*

Includes two copies of the *Facilitator Guide,* four group session videotapes, promotional/facilitator training video, *Nutrition Starter Kit,* and *Fitness Starter Kit.* When offering more than two fitness or nutrition groups simultaneously, you'll need additional *Facilitator Guides.* 0-6330-0580-0

Fit 4 *Nutrition Starter Kit*

This 12-week course includes a *Nutrition Member Workbook, Accountability Journal Refill Pack* and three-ring binder, *Wise Choices* **Fit 4** *Cookbook,* and lunch bag imprinted with **Fit 4** logo. 0-6330-0581-9

Fit 4 *Fitness Starter Kit*

A 12-week course that includes a *Fitness Member Workbook, Accountability Journal Refill Pack* and three-ring binder, the **Fit 4** *Workout* video, and exercise bag imprinted with **Fit 4** logo. 0-6330-0582-7

Fit 4 *Facilitator Guide*

Contains group session plans for facilitating both basic courses. Two copies included in *Plan Kit.* 0-6330-0588-6

Fit 4 *Accountability Journal Refill Pack*

Space to record meals and exercise activities for 13 weeks. Includes helpful nutritional and fitness information. 0-6330-0589-4

Wise Choices Fit 4 *Cookbook*

Contains easy-to-prepare recipes, menu planning suggestions, a grocery shopping list, food terms, label-reading instructions, and snack suggestions. 0-6330-0587-8

Fit 4 *Continuing Studies*

- *With All My Heart: God's Design for Emotional Wellness* 0-6330-0583-5
- *With All My Soul: God's Design for Spiritual Wellness* 0-6330-0585-1, tentatively scheduled for Summer 2001
- *With All My Mind: God's Design for Mental Wellness* 0-6330-0584-3, tentatively scheduled for Winter 2001
- *With All My Strength: God's Design for Physical Wellness* 0-6330-0586-X, tentatively scheduled for Summer 2002

Fit4.com *Web Site*

Up-to-date nutritional and fitness information, calculators for health assessments, fun quizzes, recipes, and more. Features on all four areas of wellness: emotional, spiritual, mental, and physical.

Christian Health Magazine

A great resource for balanced Christian living. Provides current health information, interesting articles about people on wellness journeys, helpful tips, recipes, biblical truths, and spiritual application to keep our lives focused on Christ. It's a great outreach tool for your church; place copies in medical offices and other businesses.

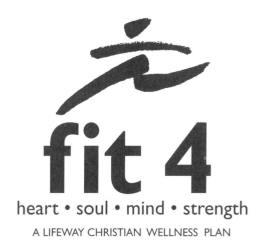

fit 4

heart • soul • mind • strength

A LIFEWAY CHRISTIAN WELLNESS PLAN

TO ORDER COPIES OF THESE RESOURCES:

Write LifeWay Church Resources Customer Service; 127 Ninth Avenue, North; Nashville, TN 37234-0113; Fax order to (615) 251-5933; Phone 1-800-458-2772; Email to *customerservice@lifeway.com;* Order online at *www.lifeway.com;* or visit the LifeWay Christian Store serving you.

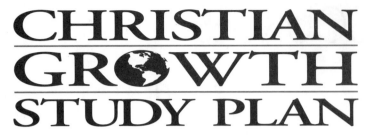

CHRISTIAN GROWTH STUDY PLAN

Preparing Christians to Serve

In the Christian Growth Study Plan (formerly Church Study Course), this book *With All My Heart* is a resource for course credit in the subject area Personal Life of the Christian Growth category of diploma plans. To receive credit, read the book, complete the learning activities, show your work to your pastor, a staff member or church leader, then complete the following information. This page may be duplicated. Send the completed page to:

Christian Growth Study Plan
127 Ninth Avenue, North, MSN 117
Nashville, TN 37234-0117
FAX: (615)251-5067
For information about the Christian Growth Study Plan, refer to the current Christian Growth Study Plan Catalog. Your church office may have a copy. If not, request a free copy from the Christian Growth Study Plan office (615/251-2525).

With All My Heart
COURSE NUMBER: CG-0535

PARTICIPANT INFORMATION

Social Security Number (USA ONLY)	Personal CGSP Number*	Date of Birth (MONTH, DAY, YEAR)

Name (First, Middle, Last)	Home Phone

Address (Street, Route, or P.O. Box)	City, State, or Province	Zip/Postal Code

CHURCH INFORMATION

Church Name

Address (Street, Route, or P.O. Box)	City, State, or Province	Zip/Postal Code

CHANGE REQUEST ONLY

☐ Former Name		
☐ Former Address	City, State, or Province	Zip/Postal Code
☐ Former Church	City, State, or Province	Zip/Postal Code

Signature of Pastor, Conference Leader, or Other Church Leader	Date

*New participants are requested but not required to give SS# and date of birth. Existing participants, please give CGSP# when using SS# for the first time. Thereafter, only one ID# is required. **Mail to:** Christian Growth Study Plan, 127 Ninth Ave., North, Nashville, TN 37234-0117. Fax: (615)251-5067

Rev. 6-99